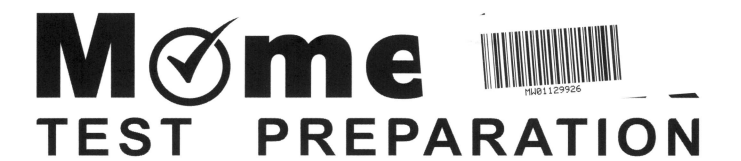

CRNI
Exam Secrets
Study Guide

DEAR FUTURE EXAM SUCCESS STORY

First of all, **THANK YOU** for purchasing Mometrix study materials!

Second, congratulations! You are one of the few determined test-takers who are committed to doing whatever it takes to excel on your exam. **You have come to the right place.** We developed these study materials with one goal in mind: to deliver you the information you need in a format that's concise and easy to use.

In addition to optimizing your guide for the content of the test, we've outlined our recommended steps for breaking down the preparation process into small, attainable goals so you can make sure you stay on track.

We've also analyzed the entire test-taking process, identifying the most common pitfalls and showing how you can overcome them and be ready for any curveball the test throws you.

Standardized testing is one of the biggest obstacles on your road to success, which only increases the importance of doing well in the high-pressure, high-stakes environment of test day. Your results on this test could have a significant impact on your future, and this guide provides the information and practical advice to help you achieve your full potential on test day.

Your success is our success

We would love to hear from you! If you would like to share the story of your exam success or if you have any questions or comments in regard to our products, please contact us at **800-673-8175** or **support@mometrix.com**.

Thanks again for your business and we wish you continued success!

Sincerely,
The Mometrix Test Preparation Team

Need more help? Check out our flashcards at:
http://mometrixflashcards.com/CRNI

TABLE OF CONTENTS

Introduction

Thank you for purchasing this resource! You have made the choice to prepare yourself for a test that could have a huge impact on your future, and this guide is designed to help you be fully ready for test day. Obviously, it's important to have a solid understanding of the test material, but you also need to be prepared for the unique environment and stressors of the test, so that you can perform to the best of your abilities.

For this purpose, the first section that appears in this guide is the **Secret Keys**. We've devoted countless hours to meticulously researching what works and what doesn't, and we've boiled down our findings to the five most impactful steps you can take to improve your performance on the test. We start at the beginning with study planning and move through the preparation process, all the way to the testing strategies that will help you get the most out of what you know when you're finally sitting in front of the test.

We recommend that you start preparing for your test as far in advance as possible. However, if you've bought this guide as a last-minute study resource and only have a few days before your test, we recommend that you skip over the first two Secret Keys since they address a long-term study plan.

If you struggle with **test anxiety**, we strongly encourage you to check out our recommendations for how you can overcome it. Test anxiety is a formidable foe, but it can be beaten, and we want to make sure you have the tools you need to defeat it.

Secret Key #1 – Plan Big, Study Small

There's a lot riding on your performance. If you want to ace this test, you're going to need to keep your skills sharp and the material fresh in your mind. You need a plan that lets you review everything you need to know while still fitting in your schedule. We'll break this strategy down into three categories.

Information Organization

Start with the information you already have: the official test outline. From this, you can make a complete list of all the concepts you need to cover before the test. Organize these concepts into groups that can be studied together, and create a list of any related vocabulary you need to learn so you can brush up on any difficult terms. You'll want to keep this vocabulary list handy once you actually start studying since you may need to add to it along the way.

Time Management

Once you have your set of study concepts, decide how to spread them out over the time you have left before the test. Break your study plan into small, clear goals so you have a manageable task for each day and know exactly what you're doing. Then just focus on one small step at a time. When you manage your time this way, you don't need to spend hours at a time studying. Studying a small block of content for a short period each day helps you retain information better and avoid stressing over how much you have left to do. You can relax knowing that you have a plan to cover everything in time. In order for this strategy to be effective though, you have to start studying early and stick to your schedule. Avoid the exhaustion and futility that comes from last-minute cramming!

Study Environment

The environment you study in has a big impact on your learning. Studying in a coffee shop, while probably more enjoyable, is not likely to be as fruitful as studying in a quiet room. It's important to keep distractions to a minimum. You're only planning to study for a short block of time, so make the most of it. Don't pause to check your phone or get up to find a snack. It's also important to **avoid multitasking**. Research has consistently shown that multitasking will make your studying dramatically less effective. Your study area should also be comfortable and well-lit so you don't have the distraction of straining your eyes or sitting on an uncomfortable chair.

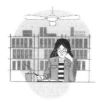 The time of day you study is also important. You want to be rested and alert. Don't wait until just before bedtime. Study when you'll be most likely to comprehend and remember. Even better, if you know what time of day your test will be, set that time aside for study. That way your brain will be used to working on that subject at that specific time and you'll have a better chance of recalling information.

Finally, it can be helpful to team up with others who are studying for the same test. Your actual studying should be done in as isolated an environment as possible, but the work of organizing the information and setting up the study plan can be divided up. In between study sessions, you can discuss with your teammates the concepts that you're all studying and quiz each other on the details. Just be sure that your teammates are as serious about the test as you are. If you find that your study time is being replaced with social time, you might need to find a new team.

2

Secret Key #2 – Make Your Studying Count

You're devoting a lot of time and effort to preparing for this test, so you want to be absolutely certain it will pay off. This means doing more than just reading the content and hoping you can remember it on test day. It's important to make every minute of study count. There are two main areas you can focus on to make your studying count.

Retention

It doesn't matter how much time you study if you can't remember the material. You need to make sure you are retaining the concepts. To check your retention of the information you're learning, try recalling it at later times with minimal prompting. Try carrying around flashcards and glance at one or two from time to time or ask a friend who's also studying for the test to quiz you.

To enhance your retention, look for ways to put the information into practice so that you can apply it rather than simply recalling it. If you're using the information in practical ways, it will be much easier to remember. Similarly, it helps to solidify a concept in your mind if you're not only reading it to yourself but also explaining it to someone else. Ask a friend to let you teach them about a concept you're a little shaky on (or speak aloud to an imaginary audience if necessary). As you try to summarize, define, give examples, and answer your friend's questions, you'll understand the concepts better and they will stay with you longer. Finally, step back for a big picture view and ask yourself how each piece of information fits with the whole subject. When you link the different concepts together and see them working together as a whole, it's easier to remember the individual components.

Finally, practice showing your work on any multi-step problems, even if you're just studying. Writing out each step you take to solve a problem will help solidify the process in your mind, and you'll be more likely to remember it during the test.

Modality

Modality simply refers to the means or method by which you study. Choosing a study modality that fits your own individual learning style is crucial. No two people learn best in exactly the same way, so it's important to know your strengths and use them to your advantage.

For example, if you learn best by visualization, focus on visualizing a concept in your mind and draw an image or a diagram. Try color-coding your notes, illustrating them, or creating symbols that will trigger your mind to recall a learned concept. If you learn best by hearing or discussing information, find a study partner who learns the same way or read aloud to yourself. Think about how to put the information in your own words. Imagine that you are giving a lecture on the topic and record yourself so you can listen to it later.

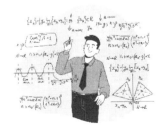

For any learning style, flashcards can be helpful. Organize the information so you can take advantage of spare moments to review. Underline key words or phrases. Use different colors for different categories. Mnemonic devices (such as creating a short list in which every item starts with the same letter) can also help with retention. Find what works best for you and use it to store the information in your mind most effectively and easily.

3

Secret Key #3 – Practice the Right Way

Your success on test day depends not only on how many hours you put into preparing, but also on whether you prepared the right way. It's good to check along the way to see if your studying is paying off. One of the most effective ways to do this is by taking practice tests to evaluate your progress. Practice tests are useful because they show exactly where you need to improve. Every time you take a practice test, pay special attention to these three groups of questions:

- The questions you got wrong
- The questions you had to guess on, even if you guessed right
- The questions you found difficult or slow to work through

This will show you exactly what your weak areas are, and where you need to devote more study time. Ask yourself why each of these questions gave you trouble. Was it because you didn't understand the material? Was it because you didn't remember the vocabulary? Do you need more repetitions on this type of question to build speed and confidence? Dig into those questions and figure out how you can strengthen your weak areas as you go back to review the material.

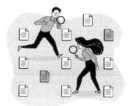 Additionally, many practice tests have a section explaining the answer choices. It can be tempting to read the explanation and think that you now have a good understanding of the concept. However, an explanation likely only covers part of the question's broader context. Even if the explanation makes perfect sense, **go back and investigate** every concept related to the question until you're positive you have a thorough understanding.

As you go along, keep in mind that the practice test is just that: practice. Memorizing these questions and answers will not be very helpful on the actual test because it is unlikely to have any of the same exact questions. If you only know the right answers to the sample questions, you won't be prepared for the real thing. **Study the concepts** until you understand them fully, and then you'll be able to answer any question that shows up on the test.

It's important to wait on the practice tests until you're ready. If you take a test on your first day of study, you may be overwhelmed by the amount of material covered and how much you need to learn. Work up to it gradually.

On test day, you'll need to be prepared for answering questions, managing your time, and using the test-taking strategies you've learned. It's a lot to balance, like a mental marathon that will have a big impact on your future. Like training for a marathon, you'll need to start slowly and work your way up. When test day arrives, you'll be ready.

Start with the strategies you've read in the first two Secret Keys—plan your course and study in the way that works best for you. If you have time, consider using multiple study resources to get different approaches to the same concepts. It can be helpful to see difficult concepts from more than one angle. Then find a good source for practice tests. Many times, the test website will suggest potential study resources or provide sample tests.

4

Practice Test Strategy

If you're able to find at least three practice tests, we recommend this strategy:

UNTIMED AND OPEN-BOOK PRACTICE

Take the first test with no time constraints and with your notes and study guide handy. Take your time and focus on applying the strategies you've learned.

TIMED AND OPEN-BOOK PRACTICE

Take the second practice test open-book as well, but set a timer and practice pacing yourself to finish in time.

TIMED AND CLOSED-BOOK PRACTICE

Take any other practice tests as if it were test day. Set a timer and put away your study materials. Sit at a table or desk in a quiet room, imagine yourself at the testing center, and answer questions as quickly and accurately as possible.

Keep repeating timed and closed-book tests on a regular basis until you run out of practice tests or it's time for the actual test. Your mind will be ready for the schedule and stress of test day, and you'll be able to focus on recalling the material you've learned.

Secret Key #4 – Pace Yourself

Once you're fully prepared for the material on the test, your biggest challenge on test day will be managing your time. Just knowing that the clock is ticking can make you panic even if you have plenty of time left. Work on pacing yourself so you can build confidence against the time constraints of the exam. Pacing is a difficult skill to master, especially in a high-pressure environment, so **practice is vital**.

Set time expectations for your pace based on how much time is available. For example, if a section has 60 questions and the time limit is 30 minutes, you know you have to average 30 seconds or less per question in order to answer them all. Although 30 seconds is the hard limit, set 25 seconds per question as your goal, so you reserve extra time to spend on harder questions. When you budget extra time for the harder questions, you no longer have any reason to stress when those questions take longer to answer.

Don't let this time expectation distract you from working through the test at a calm, steady pace, but keep it in mind so you don't spend too much time on any one question. Recognize that taking extra time on one question you don't understand may keep you from answering two that you do understand later in the test. If your time limit for a question is up and you're still not sure of the answer, mark it and move on, and come back to it later if the time and the test format allow. If the testing format doesn't allow you to return to earlier questions, just make an educated guess; then put it out of your mind and move on.

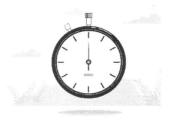

On the easier questions, be careful not to rush. It may seem wise to hurry through them so you have more time for the challenging ones, but it's not worth missing one if you know the concept and just didn't take the time to read the question fully. Work efficiently but make sure you understand the question and have looked at all of the answer choices, since more than one may seem right at first.

Even if you're paying attention to the time, you may find yourself a little behind at some point. You should speed up to get back on track, but do so wisely. Don't panic; just take a few seconds less on each question until you're caught up. Don't guess without thinking, but do look through the answer choices and eliminate any you know are wrong. If you can get down to two choices, it is often worthwhile to guess from those. Once you've chosen an answer, move on and don't dwell on any that you skipped or had to hurry through. If a question was taking too long, chances are it was one of the harder ones, so you weren't as likely to get it right anyway.

On the other hand, if you find yourself getting ahead of schedule, it may be beneficial to slow down a little. The more quickly you work, the more likely you are to make a careless mistake that will affect your score. You've budgeted time for each question, so don't be afraid to spend that time. Practice an efficient but careful pace to get the most out of the time you have.

6

Secret Key #5 – Have a Plan for Guessing

When you're taking the test, you may find yourself stuck on a question. Some of the answer choices seem better than others, but you don't see the one answer choice that is obviously correct. What do you do?

The scenario described above is very common, yet most test takers have not effectively prepared for it. Developing and practicing a plan for guessing may be one of the single most effective uses of your time as you get ready for the exam.

In developing your plan for guessing, there are three questions to address:

- When should you start the guessing process?
- How should you narrow down the choices?
- Which answer should you choose?

When to Start the Guessing Process

Unless your plan for guessing is to select C every time (which, despite its merits, is not what we recommend), you need to leave yourself enough time to apply your answer elimination strategies. Since you have a limited amount of time for each question, that means that if you're going to give yourself the best shot at guessing correctly, you have to decide quickly whether or not you will guess.

Of course, the best-case scenario is that you don't have to guess at all, so first, see if you can answer the question based on your knowledge of the subject and basic reasoning skills. Focus on the key words in the question and try to jog your memory of related topics. Give yourself a chance to bring the knowledge to mind, but once you realize that you don't have (or you can't access) the knowledge you need to answer the question, it's time to start the guessing process.

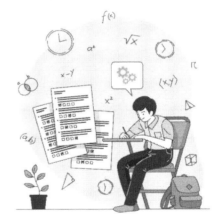

It's almost always better to start the guessing process too early than too late. It only takes a few seconds to remember something and answer the question from knowledge. Carefully eliminating wrong answer choices takes longer. Plus, going through the process of eliminating answer choices can actually help jog your memory.

Summary: Start the guessing process as soon as you decide that you can't answer the question based on your knowledge.

7

How to Narrow Down the Choices

The next chapter in this book (**Test-Taking Strategies**) includes a wide range of strategies for how to approach questions and how to look for answer choices to eliminate. You will definitely want to read those carefully, practice them, and figure out which ones work best for you. Here though, we're going to address a mindset rather than a particular strategy.

Your odds of guessing an answer correctly depend on how many options you are choosing from.

Number of options left	5	4	3	2	1
Odds of guessing correctly	20%	25%	33%	50%	100%

You can see from this chart just how valuable it is to be able to eliminate incorrect answers and make an educated guess, but there are two things that many test takers do that cause them to miss out on the benefits of guessing:

- Accidentally eliminating the correct answer
- Selecting an answer based on an impression

We'll look at the first one here, and the second one in the next section.

To avoid accidentally eliminating the correct answer, we recommend a thought exercise called **the $5 challenge**. In this challenge, you only eliminate an answer choice from contention if you are willing to bet $5 on it being wrong. Why $5? Five dollars is a small but not insignificant amount of money. It's an amount you could afford to lose but wouldn't want to throw away. And while losing

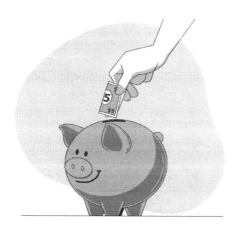

$5 once might not hurt too much, doing it twenty times will set you back $100. In the same way, each small decision you make—eliminating a choice here, guessing on a question there—won't by itself impact your score very much, but when you put them all together, they can make a big difference. By holding each answer choice elimination decision to a higher standard, you can reduce the risk of accidentally eliminating the correct answer.

The $5 challenge can also be applied in a positive sense: If you are willing to bet $5 that an answer choice *is* correct, go ahead and mark it as correct.

Summary: Only eliminate an answer choice if you are willing to bet $5 that it is wrong.

8

Which Answer to Choose

You're taking the test. You've run into a hard question and decided you'll have to guess. You've eliminated all the answer choices you're willing to bet $5 on. Now you have to pick an answer. Why do we even need to talk about this? Why can't you just pick whichever one you feel like when the time comes?

The answer to these questions is that if you don't come into the test with a plan, you'll rely on your impression to select an answer choice, and if you do that, you risk falling into a trap. The test writers know that everyone who takes their test will be guessing on some of the questions, so they intentionally write wrong answer choices to seem plausible. You still have to pick an answer though, and if the wrong answer choices are designed to look right, how can you ever be sure that you're not falling for their trap? The best solution we've found to this dilemma is to take the decision out of your hands entirely. Here is the process we recommend:

Once you've eliminated any choices that you are confident (willing to bet $5) are wrong, select the first remaining choice as your answer.

Whether you choose to select the first remaining choice, the second, or the last, the important thing is that you use some preselected standard. Using this approach guarantees that you will not be enticed into selecting an answer choice that looks right, because you are not basing your decision on how the answer choices look.

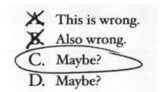

This is not meant to make you question your knowledge. Instead, it is to help you recognize the difference between your knowledge and your impressions. There's a huge difference between thinking an answer is right because of what you know, and thinking an answer is right because it looks or sounds like it should be right.

Summary: To ensure that your selection is appropriately random, make a predetermined selection from among all answer choices you have not eliminated.

Test-Taking Strategies

This section contains a list of test-taking strategies that you may find helpful as you work through the test. By taking what you know and applying logical thought, you can maximize your chances of answering any question correctly!

It is very important to realize that every question is different and every person is different: no single strategy will work on every question, and no single strategy will work for every person. That's why we've included all of them here, so you can try them out and determine which ones work best for different types of questions and which ones work best for you.

Question Strategies

⊘ READ CAREFULLY

Read the question and the answer choices carefully. Don't miss the question because you misread the terms. You have plenty of time to read each question thoroughly and make sure you understand what is being asked. Yet a happy medium must be attained, so don't waste too much time. You must read carefully and efficiently.

⊘ CONTEXTUAL CLUES

Look for contextual clues. If the question includes a word you are not familiar with, look at the immediate context for some indication of what the word might mean. Contextual clues can often give you all the information you need to decipher the meaning of an unfamiliar word. Even if you can't determine the meaning, you may be able to narrow down the possibilities enough to make a solid guess at the answer to the question.

⊘ PREFIXES

If you're having trouble with a word in the question or answer choices, try dissecting it. Take advantage of every clue that the word might include. Prefixes and suffixes can be a huge help. Usually, they allow you to determine a basic meaning. *Pre-* means before, *post-* means after, *pro-* is positive, *de-* is negative. From prefixes and suffixes, you can get an idea of the general meaning of the word and try to put it into context.

⊘ HEDGE WORDS

Watch out for critical hedge words, such as *likely, may, can, sometimes, often, almost, mostly, usually, generally, rarely,* and *sometimes.* Question writers insert these hedge phrases to cover every possibility. Often an answer choice will be wrong simply because it leaves no room for exception. Be on guard for answer choices that have definitive words such as *exactly* and *always.*

⊘ SWITCHBACK WORDS

Stay alert for *switchbacks.* These are the words and phrases frequently used to alert you to shifts in thought. The most common switchback words are *but, although,* and *however.* Others include *nevertheless, on the other hand, even though, while, in spite of, despite,* and *regardless of.* Switchback words are important to catch because they can change the direction of the question or an answer choice.

⊘ Face Value

When in doubt, use common sense. Accept the situation in the problem at face value. Don't read too much into it. These problems will not require you to make wild assumptions. If you have to go beyond creativity and warp time or space in order to have an answer choice fit the question, then you should move on and consider the other answer choices. These are normal problems rooted in reality. The applicable relationship or explanation may not be readily apparent, but it is there for you to figure out. Use your common sense to interpret anything that isn't clear.

Answer Choice Strategies

⊘ Answer Selection

The most thorough way to pick an answer choice is to identify and eliminate wrong answers until only one is left, then confirm it is the correct answer. Sometimes an answer choice may immediately seem right, but be careful. The test writers will usually put more than one reasonable answer choice on each question, so take a second to read all of them and make sure that the other choices are not equally obvious. As long as you have time left, it is better to read every answer choice than to pick the first one that looks right without checking the others.

⊘ Answer Choice Families

An answer choice family consists of two (in rare cases, three) answer choices that are very similar in construction and cannot all be true at the same time. If you see two answer choices that are direct opposites or parallels, one of them is usually the correct answer. For instance, if one answer choice says that quantity x increases and another either says that quantity x decreases (opposite) or says that quantity y increases (parallel), then those answer choices would fall into the same family. An answer choice that doesn't match the construction of the answer choice family is more likely to be incorrect. Most questions will not have answer choice families, but when they do appear, you should be prepared to recognize them.

⊘ Eliminate Answers

Eliminate answer choices as soon as you realize they are wrong, but make sure you consider all possibilities. If you are eliminating answer choices and realize that the last one you are left with is also wrong, don't panic. Start over and consider each choice again. There may be something you missed the first time that you will realize on the second pass.

⊘ Avoid Fact Traps

Don't be distracted by an answer choice that is factually true but doesn't answer the question. You are looking for the choice that answers the question. Stay focused on what the question is asking for so you don't accidentally pick an answer that is true but incorrect. Always go back to the question and make sure the answer choice you've selected actually answers the question and is not merely a true statement.

⊘ Extreme Statements

In general, you should avoid answers that put forth extreme actions as standard practice or proclaim controversial ideas as established fact. An answer choice that states the "process should be used in certain situations, if…" is much more likely to be correct than one that states the "process should be discontinued completely." The first is a calm rational statement and doesn't even make a definitive, uncompromising stance, using a hedge word *if* to provide wiggle room, whereas the second choice is far more extreme.

11

⊘ BENCHMARK

As you read through the answer choices and you come across one that seems to answer the question well, mentally select that answer choice. This is not your final answer, but it's the one that will help you evaluate the other answer choices. The one that you selected is your benchmark or standard for judging each of the other answer choices. Every other answer choice must be compared to your benchmark. That choice is correct until proven otherwise by another answer choice beating it. If you find a better answer, then that one becomes your new benchmark. Once you've decided that no other choice answers the question as well as your benchmark, you have your final answer.

⊘ PREDICT THE ANSWER

Before you even start looking at the answer choices, it is often best to try to predict the answer. When you come up with the answer on your own, it is easier to avoid distractions and traps because you will know exactly what to look for. The right answer choice is unlikely to be word-for-word what you came up with, but it should be a close match. Even if you are confident that you have the right answer, you should still take the time to read each option before moving on.

General Strategies

⊘ TOUGH QUESTIONS

If you are stumped on a problem or it appears too hard or too difficult, don't waste time. Move on! Remember though, if you can quickly check for obviously incorrect answer choices, your chances of guessing correctly are greatly improved. Before you completely give up, at least try to knock out a couple of possible answers. Eliminate what you can and then guess at the remaining answer choices before moving on.

⊘ CHECK YOUR WORK

Since you will probably not know every term listed and the answer to every question, it is important that you get credit for the ones that you do know. Don't miss any questions through careless mistakes. If at all possible, try to take a second to look back over your answer selection and make sure you've selected the correct answer choice and haven't made a costly careless mistake (such as marking an answer choice that you didn't mean to mark). This quick double check should more than pay for itself in caught mistakes for the time it costs.

⊘ PACE YOURSELF

It's easy to be overwhelmed when you're looking at a page full of questions; your mind is confused and full of random thoughts, and the clock is ticking down faster than you would like. Calm down and maintain the pace that you have set for yourself. Especially as you get down to the last few minutes of the test, don't let the small numbers on the clock make you panic. As long as you are on track by monitoring your pace, you are guaranteed to have time for each question.

⊘ DON'T RUSH

It is very easy to make errors when you are in a hurry. Maintaining a fast pace in answering questions is pointless if it makes you miss questions that you would have gotten right otherwise. Test writers like to include distracting information and wrong answers that seem right. Taking a little extra time to avoid careless mistakes can make all the difference in your test score. Find a pace that allows you to be confident in the answers that you select.

⊘ Keep Moving

Panicking will not help you pass the test, so do your best to stay calm and keep moving. Taking deep breaths and going through the answer elimination steps you practiced can help to break through a stress barrier and keep your pace.

Final Notes

The combination of a solid foundation of content knowledge and the confidence that comes from practicing your plan for applying that knowledge is the key to maximizing your performance on test day. As your foundation of content knowledge is built up and strengthened, you'll find that the strategies included in this chapter become more and more effective in helping you quickly sift through the distractions and traps of the test to isolate the correct answer.

Now that you're preparing to move forward into the test content chapters of this book, be sure to keep your goal in mind. As you read, think about how you will be able to apply this information on the test. If you've already seen sample questions for the test and you have an idea of the question format and style, try to come up with questions of your own that you can answer based on what you're reading. This will give you valuable practice applying your knowledge in the same ways you can expect to on test day.

Good luck and good studying!

Principles of Practice

Anatomy and Physiology

HEART

The **heart** is a muscle that expends energy by contraction. It is a hollow organ consisting of 4 compartments, with two different 2-sided pumps. The heart chamber called the right atrium passively receives deoxygenated blood from the body, either via the superior or inferior vena cava. After brief storage, the blood passes through the tricuspid valve, into the right ventricle, and then is ejected with positive pressure through the pulmonary valve. It then travels through the lungs by the pulmonary arteries where it becomes oxygen-rich. This oxygenated blood returns passively to the left atrium chamber of the heart via the pulmonary veins, passes through the mitral valve into the left ventricle, and is then pumped again through the aortic valve at higher pressure to other systems in the body.

HEARTBEAT

The **heartbeat** is an electrical response produced in the sinoatrial (SA) or sinus node. The sinus node is the part of the heart located at the junction between the superior vena cava (SVC), the vein that draws venous blood from the upper part of the body, and the right atrium chamber of the heart. Beats are usually generated at a rate of 60 to 100 beats per minute (bpm). The sinoatrial node is therefore the main pacemaker for the heart. Sympathetic and parasympathetic nerve fibers transmit electrical impulses to the SA.

SYSTEMIC CIRCULATION

Upon leaving the left ventricle of the heart, blood flows through the main artery of the body, the aorta. An artery is a vessel carrying blood from the heart under pressure. From the aorta, blood is carried into smaller arteries. Here the blood is bright red since it is oxygenated and it is pulsating. Arteries do not contain valves and most are located deep within tissue that is covered by muscle. Eventually these arteries terminate in smaller arterioles that form even thinner arterial capillaries. The arterial capillaries connect to venous capillaries to small veins, or venules. By this time the blood is dark because in the capillaries, an exchange of nutrients and oxygen has occurred between the blood and tissues and waste and carbon dioxide has been picked up. The venules unite to form larger veins, which eventually feed back to the heart by the superior or inferior venae cavae.

NERVE CONDUCTION IN CIRCULATORY SYSTEM

Nerve conduction is a vital component in the operation of the circulatory system. In the heart itself, there is a system of atypical muscle fibers that transmit and synchronize the electrical impulses in the heart. This is why the right and left atria contract at the same time and later both ventricles do the same. The arteries are directly stimulated through sympathetic innervation controlling the contraction and relaxation of the vessels as well as indirectly by parasympathetic innervation. These signals are transmitted by release of the hormone norepinephrine and the compound acetylcholine respectively. Veins are controlled in a similar manner.

15

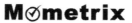

BRAIN

The **brain** is a large mass of nervous tissue that occupies the cranium or skull. It is divided into four parts, the cerebrum, cerebellum, brain stem and ventricles. The cerebrum is by far the largest part of the brain. It is divided into four lobes or hemispheres named for their adjacent bones. These lobes are the frontal lobe, which controls higher intellectual and autonomic functions; the parietal lobe, affecting position, sense, touch and motor function; the occipital lobe, or vision center; and the temporal lobe, controlling most memory and perception of sounds. The cerebellum controls movement, equilibrium, muscle tonicity, and spatial relationships. The brain stem consists of three parts, the midbrain, the pons, and the medulla oblongata; their respective functions are to transmit stimuli from the spinal cord, to relay impulses to brain centers and lower spinal centers, and to control involuntary functions. The ventricles are spaces located deep within the brain that contain cerebrospinal fluid and connect with the fluid spaces in the spinal cord.

SPINAL CORD

The **spinal cord** is a pathway to conduct impulses to and from the brain as well as a point of origin for spinal reflexes. The spinal cord consists of what is termed gray or unmyelinated matter and white or myelinated matter. The gray matter consolidates the cord's reflexes, while the white matter that surrounds it is the impulse pathway linking the spinal cord and the brain. There are separate fiber tracts that either bring these impulses to the central nervous system (ascending) or carry sensory information from the brain to the spinal cord and other neurons (descending). There are also structures that protect the spinal cord such as the vertebral column and spinous processes. Spinal ligaments help hold the spinal vertebrae together. There are also three meninges or protective membranes covering the brain and spinal cord, the pia mater, the arachnoid mater and the dura mater.

PERIPHERAL NERVOUS SYSTEM

Cranial and spinal nerves form the **peripheral nervous system**. In the brain area, there are 12 cranial nerves, which have either motor fibers, sensory fibers, or both. These nerves control voluntary muscular functions and the autonomic sensory abilities to see, hear, smell and taste. There are 31 different pairs of spinal nerves originating from different segments of the spinal cord. The cervical plexus and brachial plexus are complexes of nerve fibers supplying sensory and motor responses to the head and neck area and upper extremities respectively. Other spinal nerves include the thoracic, lumbar, sacral and cockerel nerves.

AUTONOMIC NERVOUS SYSTEM

The **autonomic nervous system** is the part of the peripheral nervous system that controls the involuntary internal functions in the body. These functions include the operation of internal organs, involuntary fibers, and glands. Portions of the hypothalamus, the brain stem and the spinal cord activate the autonomic nervous system. There are two types of nerves comprising the autonomic nervous system, sympathetic and parasympathetic. Sympathetic nerves respond to external stressors by releasing norepinephrine and transmitting impulses that increase blood pressure and heart rate and vasoconstrict peripheral blood vessels. Parasympathetic nerves operate when an individual is at rest or relaxed to maintain normal bodily functions.

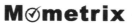

VASCULATURE

ARTERIES USED FOR VASCULAR ACCESS

There are a few **arteries** are sometimes appropriate for **vascular access**:

- The **radial artery**, which is a continuation of the brachial artery below the bend of the forearm extending to the wrist, is a site of choice. It is relatively close to the skin and if it is utilized at the wrist, it can be stabilized.
- The **ulnar artery** is larger but less superficial than the radial artery and is thus more difficult to stabilize. It is actually the terminus of the brachial artery and it extends below the elbow on the medial side of the forearm.
- The largest accessible artery is the **femoral artery**, but care must be taken to maintain dry dressings, apply digital pressure, and observe for thrombosis. The femoral artery is located halfway between the anterior superior spine of the ilium and the symphysis pubis.
- Sometimes the **pulmonary arteries** are used for vascular access. Blood can be drawn at the same time for arterial blood gases if arteries are accessed but the threat of circulatory problems or infections limit their use.

VEINS USED FOR PERIPHERAL INFUSION THERAPY

A number of **veins in the hand and forearm** can be utilized for infusion therapy. The **digital veins**, which are those along the sides of the fingers and not that widely used, combine to form three **metacarpal veins** in the hand that are often used initially. This is because for later infusions, less distal sites can be accessed without pain or inflammation. These metacarpal veins form a large vein called the **cephalic vein**, which begins in the hand and flows higher along the radial border of the forearm. The cephalic vein is an excellent choice for infusion therapy. Another choice is the **basilic vein,** which runs along the ulnar or inner side of the forearm; this is the vein that becomes prominent when the arm is flexed and bent at the elbow. Other possible choices include the **median antebrachial vein,** the **median cephalic vein**, or the **median basilic vein.** The cephalic and basilic veins extend up the arm and can sometimes be used for central intravenous therapy.

CENTRAL VEINS USED FOR CENTRAL INFUSION THERAPY

There are two different jugular or neck veins that are utilized for **central infusion therapy**, the **internal jugular vein** and the external jugular vein. The **external jugular vein** is the one easily observed on the side of the neck, and it is usually the vein of choice because of its easy access. When either jugular vein is accessed, there is a threat of air being pulled into the vascular system if the administration set becomes accidentally disconnected. The vein of choice for central vascular access devices is the subclavian vein, which is located under the collarbone. As a last resort, the health care provider could use the femoral vein.

SCALP VEINS USED FOR INFUSION THERAPY

The **scalp vein** that is most frequently utilized for infusion therapy is the **frontal (supratrochlear) vein**. This vein is on the forehead and the section running down the middle of the forehead is also called the metopic vein. In the pediatric patient, the superficial temporal vein is often used because it is easily visualized; this vein is on the side of the head and originates from a large network of veins on the scalp. Less frequently used scalp veins include the parietal vein and the occipital vein, which are found in front of and behind the ear respectively.

VEINS USED IN UNIQUE CIRCUMSTANCES FOR INFUSION THERAPY

The **umbilical vein**, which is actually located inside the umbilical cord traveling through the navel to the liver and ductus venous, is often utilized to administer infusions to newborns. There is,

17

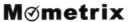

however, a high risk of septicemia using this route. In infants and children, a vein called the great saphenous vein is sometimes used for infusion. This vein runs along the medial portion of the leg originating at the ankle, and typically the lower portion above the ankle is used. The treat of thrombosis resulting in possible pulmonary emboli that can occur when using veins in the upper extremities is diminished.

INTRAOSSEOUS ADMINISTRATION

Intraosseous administration is the process of infusing right into the bone marrow. It is usually done for short periods during emergencies when an intravenous insertion proves difficult. Since the internal marrow of the bones manufactures the red blood cells, this procedure provides an indirect route. Longer bones such as the distal tibia, proximal tibia, distal femur or iliac crest are typically used. 16- to 18-gauge needles are employed, strict sterile procedures followed, and the infusion should be removed within 24 hours. Since the bones used are all in the leg or ankle, conditions such as fractured or traumatized legs, osteoporosis, or burns or cellulitis in the area contraindicate use of intraosseous administration.

AREAS TO AVOID WHEN SELECTING INFUSION SITES

In general, in adults, veins in the lower extremities should be avoided as infusion sites. This is because these veins have numerous interconnecting networks and also because they are distally located relative to the heart which makes them more susceptible to becoming inflamed, forming blood clots, or developing thrombophlebitis. Therefore, distal areas of the upper extremities are preferred. Arteries normally should only be tapped for to follow hemodynamics or to draw samples such as arterial blood gases, and not to administer medication because arterial spasm can occur which cuts off the blood supply to that area. Elderly patients often have areas of very thin skin that will not support a catheter. Areas with lesions, cellulitis, or weeping tissues should be avoided as well as injured veins. In patients who have had a mastectomy or axillary dissection, veins in those areas are generally avoided.

THERAPEUTIC PHLEBOTOMY

Phlebotomy, the removal of blood from the body, is used therapeutically to treat conditions or symptoms caused by excess red blood cells and/or iron in the blood. The most common conditions that benefit from **therapeutic phlebotomy** (also known as bloodletting) include polycythemia vera (which causes hyperviscosity of the blood due to overstimulation of bone marrow production of erythrocytes), hemochromatosis (excess iron in the blood), and porphyria cutanea tarda (which results in the accumulation of uroporphyrinogen). It is important that facility policies be followed for this procedure, including patient safety and blood disposal, in addition to following inclusion and exclusion protocols for this procedure. Generally, the blood is removed via an 18- or 20-gauge peripherally inserted catheter. Blood can be removed by gravity or using a vacutainer. Standard precautions should be followed to prevent infection.

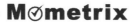

Infection Prevention and Control

LEUKOCYTES

Leukocytes are the white blood cells. They are the part of the immune system and host defense responsible for scavenging in the blood to remove foreign substances or antigens, in particular bacteria, fungi, and other infectious materials. A normal white blood cell count ranges between 4500 to 11,000 cells per cubic mm. A differential white blood cell count measures the percentages of different types of leukocytes, which all have distinct functions. The granulocytes are of two types, neutrophils and polymorphonuclear leukocytes, and they provide rapid unspecific responses to injury. When tissues are injured or inflammation occurs, a nonspecific reaction occurs which raises the granulocyte count. The agranulocytic eosinophils are cells that increase during allergic reactions or in response to parasitic infection. Both neutrophils and monocytes are macrophages, or cells that phagocytize or engulf and digest foreign particles or antigens. Lymphocytes are of two types, B and T, and they provide specific humoral (antibody) or cellular responses to bacterial or viral infections.

GRAM-NEGATIVE BACTERIA

The cell walls of **Gram-negative bacteria** are characterized by red staining. The cell wall is thinner than that of Gram-positive bacteria; however, there are two separate layers to the wall: a thin inner layer of peptidoglycan (carbohydrate polymers bound by proteins), an intervening periplasmic space, and the outer membranous layer (the lipopolysaccharide layer), which produces endotoxins, making Gram-negative bacteria extremely pathogenic. A component of the outer layer is called the S-layer; it aids in adherence and protection from pathogens. The outer layer serves to protect Gram-negative organisms from antibiotics or detergents that would disrupt the inner peptidoglycan layer and provides resistance to penicillin and other compounds. Ampicillin is able to penetrate the exterior wall although many bacteria have become resistant. Gram-negative bacteria most often associated with infusion related infections include *Acinetobacter baumannii*, *Enterobacter cloacae, Escherichia coli, Klebsiella pneumoniae, Pseudomonas. aeruginosa,* and *Stenotrophomonas maltophilia.*

GRAM-POSITIVE BACTERIA

Gram-positive bacteria are characterized by purple staining; the cell walls tend to be thicker than those of Gram-negative bacteria. About 90% of the cell wall of Gram-positive bacteria is made of peptidoglycan (carbohydrate polymers bound by proteins). The number of peptidoglycan layers varies, but there can be more than 20, making a thick-walled cell. An S-layer is attached to the peptidoglycan layer to protect the cell and aid in adherence. Gram-positive organisms tend to be easier to kill than Gram-negative because they lack the outer wall of Gram-negative organisms, and they are more sensitive to penicillin although there are resistant strains, such as methicillin-resistant *Staphylococcus aureus* (MRSA). Peptidoglycan does not occur naturally in the human body, so it is easily recognized by the immune system as an invading organism. Common Gram-positive cocci bacteria involved in infusion related infections include Coagulase-negative staphylococci, enterococci, and *staphylococcus aureus* (including MRSA).

RISK FACTORS FOR INFUSION-RELATED INFECTION

A patient can be at **increased risk for infection** during infusion therapy for a number of reasons. Many of these predisposing factors are related to the immune status including the presence of preexisting illnesses or infections, being immunodeficient or immunosuppressed, being leukopenic (low white blood cell count), or experiencing burns. If a patient has been hospitalized at length or had a number of transfusions, they are also at increased for infection. In addition, very young or

19

very old patients are more susceptible. Contamination can also occur at the healthcare site during administration.

CATHETERS INSERTION SITE RISK FACTORS

The following are sites where catheters can be inserted and unique risks or convenience factors for each:

- **Peripheral**: Catheter inserted on extremities, often the forearm. High risk of microbes at the site or poor technique of insertion by emergency team.
- **Central**: Insertion at subclavian vein under the collarbone, the jugular vein, or a femoral site such as the thigh. Very high potential for microbial growth due to warm core body temperatures at these sites. Sterile occlusive dressing is difficult to establish at the jugular and femoral sites.
- **Arterial**: Insertion into either a peripheral or pulmonary artery. Inflammation often occurs at the peripheral artery sites. Pressure must be monitored for the pulmonary catheter.
- **Intraspinal**: Catheter put in spinal column. Often associated with increased risk of infection or difficulty in maintaining a sterile dressing.
- **Intraventricular**: Introduction into one of the heart's ventricles. Increases risk for infection due to a lack of protective leukocytes there.
- **Intraosseous**: Insertion into a bony area, often as an interim measure. Can increase possibility of developing osteomyelitis.
- **Umbilical**: Catheter put in umbilical cord veins or arteries. Some risk of infection for both types.

PROBABLE SIGNS OF CATHETER-RELATED INFECTION

If **thrombophlebitis** occurs, infection might be suspected. Thrombophlebitis is the concurrent presence of inflammation and a clot. These are usually indicated by very hard veins, swelling, redness, and pain along the vein. If the tissue surrounding the site becomes discolored or drainage of pus is present, local infection can also be the source. In either case, the catheter and drainage if present should be removed and cultured before the skin is cleansed with alcohol. For thrombophlebitis alone, cold compresses are used to reduce blood flow followed by hot compresses. If infection is confirmed, antibiotic ointments, systemic therapy, and possibly surgery may be required.

FUNGAL INFECTIONS FROM INFUSION THERAPY

Fungi were originally classified as plants, but they do not produce their own food through photosynthesis and must, like animals, get the food from another source. Fungi vary widely, from one-celled microorganisms to multi-celled chains that are miles long. Fungi are used to make antibiotics, but they can also cause infection and disease. Two common classifications of fungi are molds (including mushrooms) and yeast. Fungi are not motile, but some produce spores, which can be inhaled. Some, such as the yeast *Candida albicans*, are part of the normal flora of the skin but can overgrow in an opportunistic infection, especially related to central lines and infusions. *C. albicans* accounts for about three-quarters of invasive fungal infections. As microorganisms, fungal infections can invade the sinuses, the mouth, the respiratory system, and the vagina. Antibiotics may affect the balance between bacteria and yeast, causing infection. Antifungal drugs (Amphotericin B, azoles, and flucytosine) are available, but systemic fungal infections are difficult to treat.

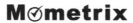

CONTAMINATION OF INTRAVENOUS FLUIDS DURING MANUFACTURING PROCESS

While production of both the intravenous fluids and the equipment used to administer them are heavily regulated by government agencies, sometimes **contamination** can occur. Very large volumes of intravenous fluids are often manufactured and sometimes stored for a long time, allowing microorganisms to grow. The healthcare provider needs to check the equipment to see if it is discolored or torn or if it has expired. The intravenous fluids themselves should be inspected to make sure they are clear with no particles, that there are no holes or cracks in the container, that the bag or bottle holds a vacuum, that the closures are not damaged, and that the expiration date is still valid. The primary causative organisms found for this type of contamination are aerobic gram-negative bacilli (a class of bacteria), and nearly all septicemias are associated with these types of bacteria. The most common specific types of causative organisms include Enterobacteriaceae species (including Serratia and Klebsiella) and Pseudomonas species.

IV SOLUTIONS AND POSSIBLE CONTAMINANTS

The type of intravenous solution utilized can contribute to the possible growth or inhibition of various microorganisms. The **most common types of intravenous solutions** and their **possible contaminants** are the following:

- **0.9% sodium chloride (NaCl)**: most bacteria will grow in this solution.
- **5% dextrose in water**: rapid growth primarily limited to the Enterobacteriaceae family, as well as *Pseudomonas cepacian.*
- **Lactated Ringer's Solution**: *Pseudomonas aeruginosa*, and a number of Enterobacter and Serratia species will grow rapidly.
- **Lipid emulsions**: most organisms, especially *Candida* species, will grow rapidly in these.
- **Crystalline amino acid and 25% dextrose solutions:** these actually inhibit most bacterial strains, but the fungus *Candida tropicalis* will grow very slowly.

PPE

PPE is the **personal protective equipment** used by nurses or other healthcare professionals to prevent dissemination of infectious agents to themselves or the patient. Types of PPE include gloves, facemasks, long-sleeved clothing and protective eyewear. Gloves should always be worn for all jobs involving exposure to blood-borne pathogenic agents when the healthcare provider is in contact with blood or bodily fluids; they can be non-sterile if insertion is at a peripheral site but otherwise sterile gloves should be worn, especially in a patient with depressed immune responses. Facemasks should be worn to protect mucous membranes or to prevent breathing onto a sterile field. Long-sleeved, usually disposable clothing provides a 2-way barrier against infectious agents. Protective eyewear, such as goggles, shields the mucous membranes of the eye.

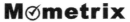

STANDARD/UNIVERSAL PRECAUTIONS

Standard or universal precautions are used with all patients to prevent the spread of pathogens. They apply to blood; all body fluids, secretions, and excretions (except sweat), regardless of whether or not they contain visible blood; non-intact skin; and mucous membranes.

- Proper handwashing should be utilized at all times.
- Wear gloves when contact is possible with any body fluids/blood.
- Never recap needles, and immediately place used needles in the closest puncture-resistant container, which should be removed for disposal when about 3/4 full. Never point a needle toward any part of the body or manipulate it using both hands.
- Should mouth-to-mouth resuscitation become necessary, it must be performed only with the use of mouthpieces, resuscitation bags, or other ventilation devices.
- A patient who contaminates the environment and will not (or cannot) follow rules of proper hygiene and environmental control must be placed in a private room.

SEPTICEMIA

Septicemia is a condition where microorganisms are actively multiplying in the bloodstream. It is more severe than transient bacteremia or viremia where bacteria or viruses are only transient or not actively multiplying. Poor hand hygiene or use of aseptic technique or failure to rotate insertion sites by the health care provider can sometimes cause this. In addition, the patient may already have microorganisms on their skin or in their system. If they are immunocompromised, often by the antimicrobial therapy they are receiving, this skin microflora can be altered or microorganisms in the gastrointestinal tract can cross over into normally sterile body tissues and the blood. Also, a catheter can become contaminated from a patient's infection at another site. The main bacterial causative agents are staphylococci primarily, coagulase-negative staphylococci species, certain Escherichia coli species, Klebsiella pneumoniae, and Pseudomonas. The fungus Candida albicans is another culprit.

DIFFERENCE BETWEEN BACTEREMIA AND SEPTICEMIA

Both **bacteremia** and **septicemia** can occur after catheter insertion. They are both basically blood stream infections related either to a primary infection caused by microorganisms migrating from the insertion site or the exacerbation of existing infections. Bacteremia merely indicates the presence of bacteria in the blood, but in the case of septicemia these bacteria are actively multiplying. Simple bacteremia can be associated with fever, chills and hypotension, but with septicemia the symptoms can progress to a rapid heartbeat, abnormally fast breathing, nausea, vomiting, diarrhea, oliguria, respiratory and vascular failure, shock and ultimately death if not recognized and treated. Septicemia can occur within a few hours after starting parenteral treatment.

SIGNS AND SYMPTOMS AND POSSIBLE CAUSES

Septicemia is a state caused by massive amounts of pathogenic bacteria in the bloodstream. The initial symptoms may be mild like fever, chills, sluggishness and headache, but these can progress to a rapid pulse, inability to stand up, flushing, backache, nausea, vomiting or hypotension. Ultimately, the vascular system can shut down and shock or even death may occur. Causes include contamination of the solution or equipment during manufacturing, storage or use; the structure or material of the catheter; translocation of microorganisms from another site such as the urinary tract, a wound or the gut; or manipulations to the system or lengthy dwell times. For example, 5% dextrose in water promotes rapid growth of some species. The protective fibrin sheath that encases and protects against infection by adherence is less effective with some materials.

22

Copyright © Mometrix Media. You have been licensed one copy of this document for personal use only. Any other reproduction or redistribution is strictly prohibited. All rights reserved.

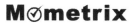

CLABSI

Intensive care patients routinely have central venous catheters placed for the administration of fluids, medications, parenteral nutrition and other supportive therapies. **Central line blood stream infections (CLABSI)** occur when a confirmed (by laboratory analysis) bloodstream infection occurs in a patient with a central line in place for greater than 2 calendar days on the date of the confirmed infection. Central line blood stream infections contribute to an increase in hospital length of stay, a marked increase in healthcare costs, and a higher mortality rate for those patients that acquire them. CLABSI is often a preventable occurrence and many evidence-based practices have been identified in their prevention. Strategies aimed at prevention of CLABSI include hand hygiene, strict aseptic technique in accessing and maintaining the catheter, thorough assessment of the catheter insertion site daily, and appropriate site care.

Signs and symptoms: Fever, chills, hypotension, tachycardia, erythema, edema and/or drainage at the catheter site, and pain/tenderness at the catheter site.

Diagnosis: CBC, blood cultures and culture of the catheter tip.

Treatment: Once the causative organism is identified, antimicrobial treatment will be initiated. The central venous catheter may also be removed.

PREVENTION OF CATHETER-RELATED INFECTIONS

The infusion nurse can aid in **preventing catheter-related infections** by maintaining impeccable hand hygiene, using good sterile technique, inspecting all equipment and dressings regularly, maintaining sterile and dry dressings at the site, rotating the insertion site, maintaining a closed sterile system, dedicating an individual line for parenteral nutrition, and following pharmacy mixing protocols. In addition, there are some more specific recommendations for types of solutions or catheter insertion sites. Blood products should be infused within a 4-hour time frame and lipid-containing nutrition solutions within 24 hours after hanging. Other types of medications or solutions should only be administered beyond 24 hours when sterile, closed and well-documented systems have been maintained and the prescribed medications or solutions have been determined to be stable for that length of time. Central venous catheters should be inserted into the distal tip of the vena cava, while peripheral arterial or pulmonary artery catheters should be disposable and replaced within about 4 days.

ANTIMICROBIAL PREPARATIONS FOR APPLICATION TO INSERTION SITE

Types of preparations is usually used to **cleanse the insertion site** and reduce exposure to microbial pathogens before putting a catheter in include the following:

- **70% isopropyl alcohol**: Denatures proteins, generally non-toxic and non-allergenic.
- **Chlorohexidine gluconate**: Binds to protein in the bacterial cell wall, antibacterial effects are long-lasting even in the presence of organic materials, yet there is virtually no systemic effect.
- **Povidone-iodine**: Crosses the cell wall and substitutes the microbial components with free iodine, can kill a wide range of agents including both gram-negative and gram-positive bacteria, fungi and yeast, but the effect can be negated by blood, serum, other proteinaceous material, or subsequent application of 70% isopropyl alcohol.
- **Acetone**: No proven reduction in rate of infection, and can cause local inflammation or skin irritation.

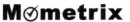

DIAGNOSTIC METHODS TO DETERMINE WHETHER AN INFECTION IS CATHETER-RELATED

Cultures can be done of the parenteral fluid, its container, the administration set, the catheter tip, the patient's blood, or swabs of the site of drainage. Normally, two blood samples would be drawn, one to isolate aerobic pathogens and another for anaerobic agents. If possible, a simple gram-stain can be done on the drainage. If catheter colonization is confirmed, then a **semi-quantitative culture** can be done after disinfecting the insertion site with 70% isopropyl alcohol, cutting the catheter, and leading fluid into a sterile container; if greater than 15 CFUs (colony forming units) are found, intravascular infection is confirmed. A **quantitative culture** can be obtained by drawing blood from two different sites, through the catheter and at a peripheral location. If the concentration of microorganisms in the catheter blood sample is at least 5 to 10 times greater than the peripheral site, catheter-related infection is confirmed and it must be removed.

ANTIMICROBIAL TREATMENT OF CATHETER-RELATED INFECTIONS

Initially, **catheter-related infection** is usually treated with some sort of broad-spectrum antimicrobial therapy in order to decrease the majority of organisms that might be present. After the actual causative agents are isolated, the therapy can be adjusted and targeted to those microorganisms. If the intravascular device remains, sometimes the antimicrobial therapy can be started through the lock system. The condition of the patient or host in terms of other disease states, renal or liver function, age, immune profile, or location of infection can influence the selection of therapeutic agent. This means that the drug selected for therapy must be considered in terms of its toxicity, possible drug interactions, cost, dose, and route and frequency of administration. Laboratory tests to monitor the concentration of the drug in the blood must be done at various intervals.

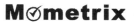

Legal/Professional Issues

CONCEPTS ASSOCIATED WITH MAINTAINING QUALITY PROGRAMS

Programs to assess and maintain **quality measures** in nursing and many other areas revolve around a number of concepts:

- One is QA, or **quality assurance**, which a method to evaluate the degree of excellence by monitoring, evaluating and correcting problems if detected.
- Another term, less used perhaps in health care than in other fields, is **total quality management**, or TQM, which involves the formulation of an organizational mission statement encompassing the goal of satisfying the client.
- Total quality improvement (TQI) and continuous quality improvement (CQI) are concepts involving a continuous process of improvement.
- Nursing (and healthcare) tends to focus more on the last concept, which is **performance improvement (PI).** PI is a leadership-driven, organizational-focused process. For healthcare professionals, this typically means developing a process to design, measure, assess, and improve performance that can have a positive effect on patients.

KNOWLEDGEABLE STAFF FOR PERFORMANCE IMPROVEMENT PROGRAMS

Any **performance improvement program** for a healthcare setting needs knowledgeable staff as a high priority. Orientation programs for nurses are mandatory including departmental policies, familiarization with specific tasks required, and any other needed education. There should be policies in place to validate the nurse's competency which typically should be evaluated once or twice a year. In addition, national certification or some sort of other credential process should be a goal, especially for any professional practicing higher level procedures. A mechanism for recertification should be included. Further, the hallmarks of successful programs also include opportunities for continuing medical education and the opportunity to do research.

PERFORMANCE STANDARDS

Performance standards are of three classifications:

- **Structural standards**, which basically outline organizational goals and policies.
- **Process standards**, guidelines focusing on the practitioner and their specific tasks and functions.
- **Outcome standards**, reflective of desired goals in regard to patient care.

Another way to look at performance standards is whether they focus on the patient (standards of care), the healthcare provider (standards of practice), or the administrative process (standards of governance). All components are needed in a healthcare setting.

SAFE ADMINISTRATION OF PARENTERAL INVESTIGATIONAL DRUGS, ANTINEOPLASTIC DRUGS, OR BLOOD COMPONENTS

Parenteral investigational drugs are only administered with informed consent and under the direction of a principal investigator on the medical staff and with prior approval of the healthcare organization. Administration of **antineoplastic therapies** requires the development of and adherence to special protocols for extravasation, spills, and vesicant drug use. In addition, the waste from these procedures is usually cytotoxic and biohazardous so latex surgical gloves should usually be worn and there should be specially designed containers and a tracking system for the waste. **Blood products** to be given in an acute setting should be used within a half hour or taken back to

25

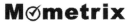

the blood bank and the patient should be closely monitored for about 15 minutes and infusion discontinued immediately if a reaction is observed.

LEGAL CLAIMS OF MEDICAL NEGLIGENCE AND MALPRACTICE

Legally, claims of negligence and malpractice are both situations that involve civil law. **Civil law** is applicable to the rights of private individuals or organizations, where there is not an offense against the general public involved. To establish a claim of **negligence**, criteria include individual propriety ownership of the duty or task, failure to meet standards, injury to the patient as a result, and proof of this breach of care. Sometimes **malpractice** could be considered the same thing as negligence, but in the case of malpractice the individual has acted negligently as part of a recognized and accountable profession with clearly defined boundaries. For nurses, the scope of their authority is clearly defined in the State Nurse Practice Act, so most negligence could be considered malpractice.

LEGAL TORTS

Legally, a **tort** is a civil offense involving a wrongful act of a private individual against another person or property. There are a number of types of torts. For example, an **assault** involves coercion or a perceived threat of such, whereas **battery** is actual physical harm. For a nurse, any physical contact without the patient's permission might be considered battery. **Coercion** is a situation in which one person forces another to act in a certain manner through threats or intimidation. **False imprisonment** is defined as putting an individual in a confined area against their will, which in a healthcare setting could mean use of restraints. Other types of torts include slander or oral defamation, libel or defamation in the media, and disclosure of private confidential information.

OBTAINING LEGALLY-BINDING INFORMED CONSENT

A patient must be sufficiently educated about their procedures and possible outcomes before freely consenting to what is known as informed consent. The patient must usually be able to authorize the consent themselves with their signature without coercion and with a witness present, but a legally recognized and approved third party can give the consent sometimes. The third party must be associated with the patient, such as the custodial parent or legal guardian of a minor. In emergency situations, a witnessed telephone call or verbal consent may be valid. Special informed consent is always required when investigational therapies are administered as part of a research study.

REGULATING BODIES ASSOCIATED WITH STANDARDS OF INFUSION NURSING CARE

On a federal level, there are two **regulating bodies** that control aspects of healthcare administration including infusion nursing.

The first is the **Food and Drug Administration (FDA),** which regulates all aspects up to the distribution of drugs, cosmetics and medical devices; faulty labeling, packaging and equipment as well as reactions or deaths upon use must be reported to the FDA.

Secondly, the **Occupational Safety and Health Administration (OSHA)** basically governs compliance with safety procedures.

The **Joint Commission** provides programs to ensure quality in healthcare organizations. Each state has a state regulatory board or **State Board of Nursing** that develops requirements for licensure and practice through their Nursing Boards of Registration and Nurse Practice Act. These can vary slightly between states. The **Infusion Nurses Society (INS)** has established their own principles for practice in their publication *Infusion Nursing Standards of Practice,* and they establish the Certified Registered Nurse Infusion (CRNI) certification.

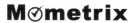

Use of Data to Understand and Institute Change in Performance Improvement Programs

There a quite a few ways **data can be collected and analyzed**, but there are a few that are more commonly applied to performance improvement within a healthcare organization. Trends can be analyzed in two ways, either as process indicators or outcome indicators. The former quantifies the proportion of times a process is completed successfully relative to the total number of times it was performed, and an outcome indicator states the number of occurrences of some action divided by the total at risk population. Both of these parameters could be considered rate-based occurrences; in other words, they express some type of proportion representative of quality of care. There are also sentinel occurrences which are unpredictable serious events that need to be investigated because there is an expected compliance rate of 100%. Expected compliance rates for rate-based occurrences are usually determined relative to benchmarks.

Access Devices

Equipment

ADMINISTRATION SETS

Some **administration sets** are designed just to deliver a single primary solution or medication. **Straight sets**, which may not have an injection port, are used for this purpose. Other types of sets permit administration of **secondary** medications or solutions, commonly referred to as **"piggyback solutions"**. There are a number of these types of sets, including the check-valve set, the secondary set, or a Y-type set. The check valve set has an integrated valve that allows a secondary solution to be injected through it and administered without cross-mixing when the height of the primary solution is lowered. The secondary set is a very short set that is attached above the check valve through a Y-configured port. The Y-type set is used with a filter or integrated hand pump. Other variations include a **controlled-volume set,** which contains a vented calibrated chamber, a retrograde set primarily used for children and neonates, and a dedicated set, which is always used with a specific device.

CONSIDERATIONS FOR ADMINISTRATION SET SELECTION

Special considerations when selecting and utilizing an administration set include:

- Some administration sets contain latex parts and should not be used for patients with latex sensitivity.
- Sets made of polyvinyl chloride cannot be used with certain medications, notably Taxol.
- The set diameter and consequent drip rate must be taken into consideration.
- The injection and access ports should be needleless and should be located beyond the drip chamber close to distal end of the set.
- Sets should be changed if contamination occurs or if any changes in the product are suspected.
- When lipid emulsions or blood products are being administered, the sets should be changed every 24 or 4 hours respectively.
- The solution should be changed as well when symptoms in the patient suggesting infection or cardiac response are observed.

CONNECTORS AND OTHER TYPES OF ADD-ON OR JUNCTION SECUREMENT DEVICES

The preferred type of **connecter** in infusion is the **Luer-Lok**. It allows an administration kit to be connected to an additional device or catheter with minimal possibility of accidental disconnections that might put the patient at risk. This is accomplished by inserting the male Luer of the administration kit into the female Luer of the other device with a locking clasp. A similar Luer slip without the locking device is not as good because it can pull apart. Add-on devices can include extension sets, stopcocks, injection or access ports for administration of intermittent or short-term therapy, devices that keep catheters in place, vented spike adaptors, caps, and other devices.

CALCULATING DROP FACTOR FOR AN ADMINISTRATION SET

The **drop factor** of the administration set (gtt/mL) must be known in order to calculate the flow rate, or drops per minute (gtt/min). Macrodrip sets typically deliver 10 to 20 gtt/mL and are employed for larger or less accurate volumes. Microdrip sets deliver 60 gtt/mL but should be used

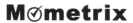

only for small volumes or careful measurements. Drops per minute (gtt/min) are calculated as follows:

Total mL x drop factor (in gtt/ml)/total minutes = gtt/min (drops per minute)

SOLUTION CONTAINERS

Solution containers are of two types:

- The first type, **glass bottles**, depends on air for flow and thus creates open systems. Because the glass bottle does not collapse as solution flows, venting is required. This necessitates the type of administration kit that allows air to enter or in some cases a vented spike adaptor is used.
- **Plastic bags** provide another type of container, which is a closed system. The plastic bag collapses during solution flow preventing exposure to the air and the possibility of air emboli. Non-vented administration sets are used with plastic bags. There are also administration sets that have dual vented/non-vented applications as the cap can be opened or kept closed.

FILTERS

Three **types of filters** often utilized in infusion therapy include the following:

- Some administration sets have filters directly uncorroborated into the design, known as **"in-line."** In this case, there is very little risk of contamination because the filter cannot separate from the set. On the other hand, these are usually located in the upper part of the set and do not filter lower add-ons and if they clog the whole set must be changed.
- An **add-on filter** can be placed anywhere, particularly at the distal end of the set, which is preferable, and it can be easily changed if clogged or defective. However, it can become separated from the administration set.
- Sometimes, if a medication is to be given as a large single dose, a **filter needle** that may retain particles from 1 to 5 microns in size may be utilized.

STRUCTURAL AND RETENTIVE PROPERTIES OF DIFFERENT FILTER TYPES

Membrane filters are screen-type filters possessing uniformly sized pores or holes. They keep any particle larger than the pore size on the membrane, and thus they are usually the type of filter used to retain and filter out bacteria, fungi, or unique contaminants. The 0.2-micron pore size is routinely used to filter bacteria out of intravenous solutions. It should not be utilized for blood products, lipids, intravenous push, or with some medications. Larger filters with pore sizes of 1 or 5 microns filter out particulate matter. A special size of 1.2 microns is generally used to administer total nutrition admixtures. Other types of filters are called **depth filters,** consisting of irregularly sized fibers and used to filter particulates only, and hollow fiber filters, which are made of fibers that withstand high pressure.

ADMINISTRATION OF BLOOD PRODUCTS

Blood filters are integrated right into some administration sets and are designed to remove either particulate matter or specific blood components from the blood or its components. Standard blood filters have a much bigger pore size than those used for intravenous solutions, ranging from 170 to 260 microns. Microaggregate blood filters have a smaller pore size of only 20 to 40 microns and are really only used during heart bypass surgery or for repeated transfusions because their small pore size slows the flow rate. There are also two types of leukocyte-reduction filters available, one that removes leukocytes from red blood cells and another that removes leukocytes from platelets.

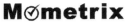

CLASSES OF ELECTRONIC INFUSION DEVICES

Electronic infusion devices are either controllers or positive-pressure infusion pumps:

- A **controller** is an electronically controlled device that dispenses fluids merely by the aid of gravity. A desired flow rate is set on the device and the tubing pressure is regulated by counting the drops. In this case, the solution must be placed about 3 feet above the catheter insertion site to aid gravity.
- Another type of device, the **positive-pressure infusion pump** actually exerts pressure to circumvent resistance. It is used to administer medications especially complex therapies, when large volumes are given, or when great attention is necessary since these pumps should be more accurate. The average pressure delivered is about 5 to 10 pounds per square inch (psi).

PUMPS FOR DISPENSING MEDICATION AND SOLUTIONS

There are several mechanisms to systematically deliver medications or solutions. One type, the **volumetric pump**, measures the volume of fluid displaced into a container attached to the administration set. The mechanism of action could be either use of a syringe to withdraw and then push solution through the set, a linear peristaltic pump which compresses tubing to push the solution, or sequential filling and emptying of small reservoirs. A syringe pump is ideal for infants or other situations where small and/or intermittent amounts need to be delivered; typically, analgesics or antibiotics are given by this method. A pump employing a piston to control the solution flow operated by battery or electricity allows continuous, intermittent, or simultaneous delivery. Often, a drop sensor to count the drops as they flow is used at the same time.

DRUG LIBRARY

A **Drug Library** is a library of information incorporated into some flow control devices. This library contains information about different medications including upper and lower limits of allowed. In this way, errors in dispensing medications at the bedside can be prevented. Strict and more lax limits are usually programmed, and there are ways to bypass the stricter limits of dosage provided. This is just one precaution provided on these flow control devices. Others include a variety of alarms and controls. One essential feature is a device that has an automatic anti-free flow feature, which means that when the door is opened or the administration set is removed, a mechanical clamp prevents the flow.

MECHANICAL INFUSION DEVICES

Mechanical infusion devices are typically used for home infusion therapy. For example, one type is the elastomer balloon, usually used to infuse antibiotics or small amounts of parenteral nutrition. This device consists of a balloon inside a rigid clear container. The medication is injected into the balloon through a tamper-proof port and then ejected through an outlet port into an administration set. Another home infusion tool is a **spring-coil container** that delivers medication. A third device is a **piston syringe** that is driven by a spring-coil mechanism to deliver medications or solutions.

VEIN LOCATION DEVICES FOR INFUSION THERAPY

Finding veins to access can be difficult for patients with small or very fragile veins (such as children and older adults). Vessels should be 2 to 3 times the diameter of a catheter, so **transillumination**

devices help to locate appropriate sites for placement. Two different types of devices help to identify the position and size of veins:

- **Transillumination:** These devices, such as the Venoscope® and Transillumination Vein Locator®, utilize high intensity LED lights in a handheld device. The lights illuminate and shine through the subcutaneous tissue, allowing visualization of the veins. While still illuminated, the vein can be anchored by the nurse to prevent rolling before needle insertion.
- **Ultrasound:** Ultrasound-guided peripheral IV (USGPIV) placement is utilized for difficult to access veins, such as in patients with hypovolemia, severe edema, obesity, or scarred vessels. The probe should be covered with a sterile transparent dressing before applying sterile gel. The vein may be located with or without a tourniquet in place. The vein and the needle are tracked on a monitor, which can guide insertion into the vein.

TIP LOCATING SYSTEM

A **tip locating system** is used to verify the correct placement of the tip of a central catheter, which should be at the junction of the superior vena cava and the right atrium. The tip should always be verified prior to any infusions. Tip locating systems include:

- **Chest X-ray:** This is used not only to identify the tip of the central line to ensure it is the correct position but also to note any indications of complications, such as pneumothorax and subcutaneous emphysema. However, chest X-rays are not 100% accurate in ensuring proper placement.
- **Transesophageal echocardiogram**: TEE may be used to guide insertion of the central line and to verify placement because it clearly shows the superior vena cava and right atrial junction. This technique is most often used with central line placement prior to cardiac surgery.
- **Ultrasound**: Verifying tip location with ultrasonography may be superior to chest X-ray and is faster in emergent situations and better at identifying pneumothorax. A saline flush is used to help detect catheter position. A delay in appearance of bubbles in the heart (>2 seconds) may indicate distal location (such as in the subclavian vein).

BLOOD/FLUID WARMER AND PRESSURE CUFF

A **blood/fluid warmer** is a device that heats either solutions or blood products to a consistent temperature between 32 and 37°C. This device is most commonly used in transfusion therapy for patients with cold agglutinins, neonatal or pediatric exchange transfusions, or for large-scale rapid transfusions to avoid cardiac arrest. In patients with hypothermia or when fluids have been refrigerated, the device is sometimes used for fluid therapy as well. A pressure cuff is a sleeve that fits around a blood bag. A pressure manometer is inserted inside the cuff to cause the blood to drip more rapidly.

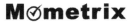

Infusion Access Devices

PERIPHERAL CATHETERS

Peripheral catheters can be made of Teflon, polyvinylchloride, polyurethane, or silicone. Silicone is the least likely to cause blood clots, giving it an advantage, whereas Teflon has the most thrombogenic potential. Some catheters are coated with heparin to reduce this possibility of inflaming the veins. Radiopaque catheters that can be seen by radiography if they break are preferred. Catheters are available in different gauges or interior size of the lumen. Types of available peripheral catheters include over-the-needle catheters, which have a needle inside; through-the-needle catheters, where the catheter is threaded through a needle into the vein; double-lumen catheters, with two entry points; and lastly midline catheters, 3 to 8 inches in length, which are generally inserted into vessels of the upper arm.

SHORT PERIPHERAL CATHETER

Short peripheral catheters are usually inserted into the hand, wrist or forearm (avoiding areas of flexion). Most are made of polyurethane. Antecubital areas are usually avoided if possible so these sites can be saved for blood draws. SPCs are used when infusions are needed for a few days, with 96 hours usually the maximum duration of the SPC. Leaving the SPC in place for longer periods increases the risk of phlebitis. Fluids include isotonic fluids/drug and fluids with pH ranging from >5 to <9m. Vesicants and IV solution with >10% glucose should be avoided. SPCs are usually over-the-needle catheters with the catheter length 7.5 cm. Gauges range from 15 (massive trauma) to 24 (small, fragile vessels). Insertion is done with sterile technique. Procedure:

- Identify target vein and insertion site, with vascular access device if necessary.
- Cleanse skin with appropriate antiseptic, such as 2% chlorhexidine in 70% isopropyl alcohol.
- Administer local anesthetic if utilizing.
- Insert catheter and look for blood return. Gauge 20 used for multipurpose medications and infusions, 22 for most chemotherapy, and 18 for multiple transfusions.
- Stabilize catheter flush with skin.
- Apply transparent semipermeable dressing.
- Catheter flushed with ≥2 mL NS every 12 hours if not in use.

MIDLINE PERIPHERAL CATHETER

Midline peripheral catheters range from 7.5 cm to 20 cm in length and may stay in place from two to four weeks. The MPC is inserted into the basilic, brachial, or cephalic veins, either 3-5 cm above or 1-2 cm below the antecubital fossa, and feeds into larger veins than the short peripheral catheter. MPCs may have single or double lumens and may be made of silicone and polyurethane materials. The tip of the catheter should be located below the axilla. Fluids include isotonic fluids/drug and fluids with pH ranging from >5 to <9m. Vesicants and IV solution with >10% glucose should be avoided. Insertion is done with sterile technique. Procedure:

- Locate target vein. A vein locator, such as transillumination device, should be used.
- Cleanse skin with appropriate antiseptic, such as 2% chlorhexidine in 70% isopropyl alcohol.
- Administer local anesthetic if utilizing.
- Insert catheter and look for blood return. Ultrasound probe may be used to ensure that the needle is properly placed before advancing the catheter. Make sure tip is not advanced beyond distal axillary vein.

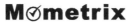

- Stabilize catheter flush with skin (suturing not generally necessary).
- Apply transparent semipermeable dressing.
- Flush every 8 to 12 hours with 10 mL saline with or without 3 mL (10 U/mL) heparin or prefilled 10 mL heparin syringe if not in use.

PERIPHERAL CATHETER INSERTION

The health care professional should wash their hands before preparation of a peripheral catheter site, and during the venipuncture they should wear gloves as well as goggles and a gown if they expect splashing. The insertion site should be prepared first by clipping off excess hair, cleaning with soap and water if necessary, and then applying an approved antimicrobial solution to the site in a circular pattern radiating outward from the expected location. Approved solutions include 2% tincture of iodine, 10% povidone-iodine, alcohol and chlorhexidine. Dilation techniques such as pumping the fist, tapping the vein, keeping the limb or other site below the heart level, or heat application are usually employed. A tourniquet should be applied 4 to 6 inches above the expected venous site only if necessary because it can cause bleeding. The actual venipuncture might be by direct insertion or indirect insertion under the skin with relocation of the vein for insertion. The stylet bevel is usually facing up so as to cause less trauma but sometimes it is inserted facing down in small veins to prevent bleeding into the surrounding tissue. Another way is to use the Seldinger technique where a guide is used to thread a catheter through a needle.

CENTRAL VASCULAR ACCESS DEVICES

Central vascular access devices or catheters can be inserted by direct venipuncture into the vein, typically either the subclavian or jugular veins. This is usually done for short-term infusions. If a catheter is indicated for long-term use, for example for 1 to 2 years, a physician may insert what is known as a tunneled catheter. This device is implanted by creating a tunnel under the skin from the vein entry point to an exit point along the chest wall. Sometimes a catheter is placed in the subclavian vein and surgically implanted under the skin. Catheters peripherally inserted into veins in the arm can also be threaded into the superior vena cava, providing central vascular system access. Only needleless devices should be used.

TUNNELED AND NON-TUNNELED CENTRAL VENOUS CATHETERS

Central venous catheters are used for long-term vascular access to administer fluids and drugs, to monitor CV pressure, and to draw blood. Central catheters may have one to three lumens, depending on the type and purpose of the catheter. Two primary types of CVCs include the following:

- **Non-tunneled catheters** are inserted percutaneously into right (or left) internal jugular vein, subclavian vein, or femoral vein. Peripherally inserted central catheters (PICCS) (one type of non-tunneled catheter) are inserted into the basilic, cephalic, or brachial vein and advanced to the superior vena cava. Non-tunneled catheters are inserted using sterile technique and local anesthetic. The catheter is secured with transparent semipermeable dressing or suture and flushed with NS after use or once a week.
- **Tunneled catheters** usually are inserted between the nipple and the sternum under the skin and into the superior vena cava and have a Dacron cuff about 5 cm from the exit point. This cuff anchors the catheter to fibrous tissue and helps to prevent migration of bacteria. Tunneled catheters are more stable for long-term therapy than non-tunneled and less prone to infection. Inserted as a surgical procedure under local or general anesthesia and flushed with NS after use or once a week.

33

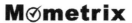

IMPLANTED PORTS

Ports that can only be implanted by a physician are usually used when either the expected duration of infusion is lengthy or for spinal catheters. When lengthy infusions of over a year are done, a single- or double-lumen catheter is inserted into the subclavian or jugular vein and connected into the vena cava. The device typically is protected by plastic, stainless steel or titanium around it. If spinal access is needed for pain management into the epidural or intrathecal space, a similar catheter is inserted into those spaces and threaded through the skin into a pocket for the port in the subcutaneous layer.

PICC LINE INSERTION

A **PICC** is a **peripherally inserted central catheter**. Extra sterile surgical precautions are necessary for this procedure including a 5-minute hand to elbow scrub with iodine-based or chlorhexidine solution, mask, cap, sterile gown, gloves, and usually goggles. The area should be surrounded by large sterile drapes and sterile towel used. PICC involves inserting the catheter into a distal vessel and then threading it into the vena cava. Preparation is similar for a central insertion into the subclavian, jugular or femoral veins or a percutaneously inserted central line. In addition, the patient should be placed either in the Trendelenburg position, which means the head lower than the feet, or in a supine position.

DRESSING CENTRAL LINE AFTER INSERTION

Once the central venous catheter is inserted and advanced to the appropriate position (junction of the superior vena cava and right atrium) and blood return assessed in all ports, all ports are flushed, sterile caps are applied to all hubs, and insertion length is verified and adjusted. Next, a catheter securing device is placed over tube at insertion site. The catheter secure device is then sutured in place if indicated, and a **sterile dressing** is applied using sterile technique:

- Lift the sterile drape that was in place for insertion and pull it back to fully expose the insertion site if necessary.
- Apply a BIOPATCH® protective disk about the catheter (underneath catheter secure device) and between sutures to provide some cushioning.
- Cleanse a three-inch area about the insertion site with a ChloraPrep® swab and let air dry.
- Apply sterile transparent semipermeable dressing, with the hub at the center of the dressing.
- Remove all drapes.

DRESSING CHANGES FOR CENTRAL LINE

Central line dressings are usually changed routinely once a week unless otherwise indicated. Protocols may vary slightly:

- Position patient with head of bed elevated and head turned away from the side that has the catheter to prevent contamination of site. The patient should wear a mask if coughing.
- Prepare sterile field and open dressing.
- Apply sterile mask and clean gloves.
- Remove old dressing by gently loosening and pulling in the direction of catheter end, avoiding any contact with skin within 7.5 cm of insertion site.
- Replace clean gloves with sterile gloves.
- Cleanse site with antiseptic (alcohol or betadine) with swab in circular motion from insertion site outward. Repeat with second swab.
- Cleanse port and first few inches of tubing with third swab.

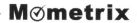

- Cleanse 3-inch area about insertion site in back and forth motion with ChloraPrep® swab.
- After antiseptic dries, apply BIOPATCH® and transparent semipermeable dressing with insertion site at center.
- Label time and date on tape and place over one end of dressing.

Nonvascular Access Options

Subcutaneous Infusion

Subcutaneous infusion (AKA hypodermoclysis) is used primarily to treat mild to moderate dehydration and to provide fluid or nutritional support for those with difficult intravenous access, such as palliative care patients, those with fragile or rolling veins, and patients who are restless or confused. It is most often used in the elderly. Sites most commonly used include the abdomen (lateral aspects), thighs, interscapular area, and upper arms, but the site selected should be one that is least likely to be disturbed by patient activities. The site selected should have adequate subcutaneous tissue (verified by pinching the tissue) and adequate skin turgor to allow for absorption of fluids. Cannulas with 22- to 24-gauge needles are inserted at 45° angle in a proximal direction into subcutaneous tissue and secured with a transparent semipermeable dressing. NS is most frequently used but other fluids may be administered as well. Hyaluronidase added to the fluid aids absorption.

Intraspinal Infusion

Intraspinal infusion includes administration into the intrathecal (subarachnoid) space directly into the cerebrospinal fluid or into the epidural space to the area next to the spinal sac, usually with insertion in the lumbar area. When possible, the catheter should be inserted below the spinal cord (L1 to L2) to prevent neurological damage. Intraspinal infusions are used primarily to control severe pain and, if successful, an infusion pump can be surgically inserted under the skin for long term analgesia. The pump contains a reservoir that is refilled about every 6 months. Intraspinal infusions may also be used to deliver chemotherapy and medications, such as baclofen, to control spasticity. Postoperative epidural infusions are often used for limited periods to control labor pain and postoperative pain. Once a spinal catheter is in place, it should be secured with a transparent semipermeable dressing. The dressing is usually changed only weekly to avoid dislodging the catheter and reduce risk of infection.

Intraosseous Infusion

Intraosseous (IO) infusion is an alternative to IV access for neonates, pediatric emergencies, and adult emergencies when rapid temporary access is necessary or when peripheral or vascular access can't be achieved. It is often used in pediatric cardiac arrest. Because yellow marrow replaces red marrow, access in those over 5 is more difficult. Preferred sites include:

- 0-5: Proximal tibia (preferred).
- Older children and adults: medial malleolus. The sternum can support higher infusion rates. Other sites include the distal femur, clavicle, humerus, and ileum.

IO infusion is used to administer fluids and anesthesia and to obtain blood samples. Equipment requires a special needle (13-20 gauge) as standard needles may bend. The bone injection gun (BIG) with a loaded spring facilitates insertion. The FAST needle is intended for use in the sternum of adults and prevents accidental puncture of the thoracic cavity. Knowledge of bony landmarks and correct insertion angle and site are important. Position is confirmed by aspiration of 5-10 mL of blood and marrow before infusion. Special stabilizer dressings with a cup about the needle are applied to keep the needle in position.

Special Populations

PREMATURE NEONATE

A **premature neonate**, also referred to as a preterm or premature infant, is one that is born less than 37 weeks after conception at the time of delivery. Special care is really needed to maintain fluid and electrolyte balance in these premature neonates because very rapid changes in the total body water distribution takes place at birth. In addition, the actual gestational age is important to consider. The total body water and extracellular fluid (ECF) are at higher percentages at lower gestational ages. As the fetus grows, the proportion of the ECF diminishes while the intracellular fluid (ICF) and the portions of the cells increase.

UNIQUE CHARACTERISTICS THAT AFFECT CARE

The **body surface area,** or BSA, of premature neonates is about five times greater than their body weight which means that a lot of water can be lost, including through the stomach and intestines. In addition, they have increased metabolic waste to excrete and fewer ways available to buffer and maintain a normal pH. The neonate's kidneys and renal functions are not fully developed. The skin is thin, fragile, and unstable. Their liver is unable to perform functions like metabolizing drugs, form plasma proteins and the like. Their ability to generate heat is diminished which means the healthcare worker needs to keep them warm. Some electrolytes are relatively high while others are relatively reduced.

NEONATE

A **neonate** is defined as an infant born at full term to about 4 weeks after their birth. The body water content of a full-term neonate is approximately three-quarters of their total body weight. Almost half of that water is in the extracellular fluid compartment. Blood in the circulation is at levels of approximately 85 to 90 mL per kg body weight. The relative body surface area is still much greater than that of an adult. The neonate may have a low pH. As in the premature neonate, bodily functions such as renal, hepatic, thermoregulatory, and electrolyte balance functions are still immature. Full-term neonates regulate heat better than a premature infant.

PSYCHOSOCIAL CONSIDERATIONS WHEN CARING FOR NEONATES

Neonates, whether premature or not, are very susceptible to stress, so supportive measures such as using a pacifier, talking softly, minimizing sudden movements or wrapping them should be undertaken. They need to be kept warm and their pain needs to be managed. To avoid vomiting, procedures should be performed either before they are fed or quite a while thereafter. If they do become stressed, their oxygen consumption is increased and they can develop cardiovascular side effects.

INFANT VERSUS TODDLER

An **infant** is generally defined as up to 1 year old whereas the term **toddler** refers to period from 1 to 3 years old. The approximate total body water content (TBW) decreases during infancy, and the extracellular fluid decreases dramatically during that first year. By the end of their second year, a toddler's TBW approaches that of an adult. An infant still has a proportionately larger body surface area than an adult, but by the end of their third year a toddler's BSA is proportionately similar to an adult. Acid-base regulation and normal pH (7.35 to 7.45) are achieved by the time the child is considered an infant, but other systems remain immature until they are a toddler. Serum phosphate levels are abnormally high until about 5 years of age.

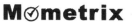

Social and Emotional Needs of Children from Infancy to Adolescence

When a child is an infant, his or her major fears are primarily separation and apprehension when exposed to strangers; they either trust or mistrust individuals. By about 3 to 6 months, they can recognize and pinpoint pain. In addition to separation anxiety, a toddler wants to be in control and is thinking primarily of himself. They are increasingly mobile and want their independence. A preschooler, defined as 3 to 6 years of age, has usually developed a more defined sense of independence and a willingness to please others. They still have fears such as bodily injury, losing control, or the unknown. By school age, defined as 6 to 12 years of age, they are increasingly independent and private. They have more mature needs, such as developing self-esteem, helping others, and following directions. An adolescent, at 12 to 18 years old, is pretty much able to think abstractly, reason, and accept increasing amounts of responsibility. They are also very conscious of their image, can experience mood swings, and often have trouble complying with authority figures.

Patient History for Younger Children

A myriad of questions should be included on a **patient history**. Until the child is old enough to answer, a parent or caregiver should be relaying this information. If a child is younger than 2 years or developmentally disabled, or was premature, some unique questions should be included. These questions address the history of the mother prior to the birth, the genesis of the labor and delivery including Apgar scores and complications if any, the number of weeks between conception and birth, birth weight and length, and presence of any inherited diseases or neonatal illnesses.

A **pediatric patient history** alone can help diagnose the majority of childhood medical conditions. This history should include questions about how their health status has been managed; their means of nutrition and any feeding problems, including how they are being fed (if infants); difficulties such as chocking, cyanosis, and presence of vomiting; their medication history; presence of allergies; their patterns and problems with either bowel or bladder voiding; skin quality; and family history. In addition, perception or social issues should be addressed such as their patterns of activity and exercise, sensory perception deficits, how they perceive themselves, and abilities to communicate and cope.

Measuring Height and Weight During Pediatric Physical Examination

For a child younger than 24 months, the patient lies down and their **height** from crown to heel is measured. Starting at about age 2 years, the standing height or stature can be measured. Infants should be weighed without clothes on a platform type of scale. A **daily weight** under similar circumstances should be obtained for an infant undergoing infusion therapy. A standing scale is used for toddlers and older children. Measurements should be taken with as little clothing as possible and recorded to the nearest one-quarter pound. Changes need to be monitored closely as weight loss generally indicates fluid volume changes and can lead to dehydration.

Pediatric Patient's Temperature

Temperature can be measured with a mercury thermometer, but because mercury is toxic, alternative devices are often used these days especially in pediatric patients. These alternative devices include electronic thermometers to be used in the armpit, oral or rectal areas, tympanic membrane sensors, disposable strips, or digital thermometers. Normal rectal temperatures range on either side of 37°C, but since taking these risks rectal wall perforation, they are not routinely done today. Instead, axillary (armpit) or oral measurements are more common and the normal values expected are a little lower, up to 37°C. Ages for these are typically older too, at least 4 years or 2 years old respectively. The tympanic membrane sensor usually is too big for the ear canal until the child is a year old. Observing an abnormal temperature can indicate sepsis (low) or dehydration (high early but may become subnormal).

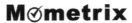

TAKING A CHILD'S PULSE

In a younger child of less than 2 years, the best place to take their **pulse** is the apical pulse for an entire minute. The radial pulse can be used for older children. The average normal pulse rate decreases with age. In a neonate or infant, the normal range is 120 to 160 beats per minute. This decreases to only 60 to 90 beats per minute by adolescence. If the pulse rate is abnormal or the rhythm changes, fluid volume or electrolyte imbalances are usually the cause. Distal pulses such as the femoral pulse should also be taken in healthy children in addition to the radial pulse because discrepancies between the two can indicate constriction of the blood vessels and a variety of other complications.

RESPIRATORY RATES AND BLOOD PRESSURE MEASUREMENTS IN PEDIATRIC PATIENTS

The **respiration rate,** or number of respirations per minute, in pediatric individuals decreases as they progress from infancy to adolescence. The respiratory rate in an infant should be between 30 and 60 breaths a minute whereas by the time the child is an adolescent, their rate should be between 12 and 16 breaths a minute. Rhythm and depth of the breath should also be observed, and any period of 15 seconds or longer without a respiration, known as apnea, should be noted. In a child, blood pressure tends to increase slightly with age. For example, in infants, the systolic pressure (which measures pressure upon heart contraction) is normally 74 to 100 mm Hg (mercury) and the diastolic pressure (at relaxation or expansion) typically 50 to 70 mm Hg. By adolescence, normal values would be a systolic pressure of 94 to 140 mm Hg and a diastolic pressure of 62 to 88 mm Hg.

MEASURING FLUID VOLUME DEFICIT IN CHILDREN

Observation of several different mucous membranes can give an **indication of fluid volume deficit**. These membranes include those in the mouth, particularly between the cheek and the gums, where dry mouth may be observed. The tongue may be small if a child is not properly hydrated. They may not experience tearing. In infants, the soft spot on the baby's head can be sunken or depressed if the child is dehydrated. On the other hand, a bulging spot or fontanel can indicate fluid excess or other conditions such as intracranial pressure or hydrocephalus. Urine excretion should be measured in milliliters per kilogram per hour. A less reliable measurement would be urine specific gravity. Neurological changes can also indicate fluid or electrolyte imbalance.

ASSESSING PEDIATRIC SKIN CONDITION

The health care provider should observe the **pediatric patient's skin** in a number of ways. The skin color usually is best observed at the eyeball, nail beds, ear lobes, lips, oral membranes, palms or soles of the feet. It can be used in a number of differential diagnoses including anemia (pale color) and liver disease (jaundice). The presence of cyanosis, or abnormally bluish skin, can be associated with hypoxia but often is normal in newborns. The skin should also be observed for its temperature, its amount of elasticity, presence of edema, and rate of capillary refill. Turgor measurements are one of the best indications of whether the child is getting adequate fluid levels and nutrition.

NORMAL SERUM ELECTROLYTE LEVELS IN CHILDREN

Levels of several cation type **electrolytes** as well as bicarbonate may be slightly low for preterm or full-term neonates. Phosphorus and phosphate levels are actually slightly higher in that population. By the fortieth week of gestation, adult sodium levels are achieved, about 140 mEq/L. By the time a child is about a week and a half old, they have potassium levels averaging 5 mEq/L. A week-old neonate usually has calcium levels approaching those of an adult, which should be 8.7 to 10.3

mg/dL by one month. Chloride levels are generally 99 to 111 mEq/L and magnesium concentration is 1.3 to 2.1 mEq/L, similar to adults. Preterm neonates should have a phosphorus/phosphate concentration of between 5.6 and 11.7 mg/dL, which keeps decreasing with age to 2.5 to 4.5 mg/dL in adolescence.

INTERRELATED LABORATORY VALUES FOR HEMOGLOBIN, HEMATOCRIT, AND BILIRUBIN

Hemoglobin is the iron-containing substance in red blood cells that combines with oxygen to transport the latter from the blood to the tissues. Infants grow rapidly with a concurrent increase in blood volume and low hemoglobin levels of about 9 to 14 g/dL at age 6 months. By 12 years of age, there is generally a little higher concentration of hemoglobin in males than females. At that time, normal values are 13.5 to 18 g/dL for males, 12.0 to 16.0 g/dL for females. The **hematocrit** indicates the percentage of the blood that consists of red blood cells, which is the highest in neonates (45% to 65%). By adolescence, values are equivalent to those in adults, 44% to 52% for males, 39% to 47% for females. **Bilirubin** is a product of hemoglobin metabolism, which is normally high in neonates, and should be about 0.1 to 0.7 mg/dL by age 1 month. The unconjugated form of bilirubin can accumulate in the brain and cause irreparable damage so high levels above 12 should be noted and treated with phototherapy.

LABORATORY TESTS EVALUATING FLUID AND ELECTROLYTE BALANCE IN CHILDREN

Other **laboratory tests** that are usually ordered **to evaluate fluid and electrolyte balance** include serum osmolality, blood urea nitrogen (BUN), serum and urine glucose levels, and arterial blood gases. BUN is important because it usually increases with fluid volume deficit; normal values increase from about 4 to 12 mg/dL in the neonate to 10 to 20 mg/dL in children above than 2 years of age. Presence of glucose in the urine can indicate severe infection. Taking arterial blood gases is the best way to evaluate the acid-base balance and look at the amount of oxygen in the blood. Arterial blood gas measurements include pH, which should be an adult value of pH 7.35 to 7.45 by age 1 month; PaO_2 which measures the amount of oxygen the lungs are delivering to the blood in mm Hg (mercury), which increases with age to 80 to 110 mm Hg by age 2 years; and $PaCO_2$ for the assessment of carbon dioxide elimination in the lungs, normal value 35 to 45 mm Hg by age 2 years. Oxygen saturation should approach 100%.

PEDIATRIC PATIENTS AND FLUID VOLUME IMBALANCES

Proportionately, a pediatric patient has more extracellular fluid relative to body size, a larger relative body surface area, immature kidneys, less homeostatic buffering capacity, and an increased metabolic rate relative to adults. These factors make rapid fluid volume replacement important. Initially, crystalloid solutions, notably Ringer's lactate, should be infused to replace the vascular fluid volume. If shock occurs, additional amounts are necessary. Then during the second phase, typically up to a day after the incident, maintenance therapy is started, and by the third phase of early recovery, generally 1 to 3 days after observation, the goal is to slowly correct any remaining imbalances.

CATHETERS USED IN NEONATES AND YOUNG CHILDREN

In neonates, **umbilical catheters** are employed. These catheters are flexible but solid-walled devices visible on radiographs that are inserted into either an umbilical artery or vein. Insertion can only be done by physician or RN trained in the technique. The umbilical venous catheter (UVC) would be temporarily inserted into the inferior vena cava below the level of the left atrium. An umbilical arterial catheter is sometimes inserted into the descending aorta but should be used cautiously because drugs are directly introduced into some major arteries. **Intraosseous catheters** are often used for emergency access in young children if a normal intravenous route cannot be found. In this case, the needle is inserted into the medullary cavity of a lengthy bone.

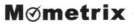

CONSIDERATIONS FOR VENIPUNCTURE SITES IN CHILDREN

In a child, many of the same sites as adults are used for **venipuncture**. However, some sites may be more or less available in a child. For peripheral catheters, lower extremities are often used if the child does not walk yet, especially portions of the foot as they can be easily palpitated and observed. In the upper extremities, the dorsal venous network in the hand is difficult to use because infants have an excessive amount of subcutaneous tissue and the digital veins also infiltrate easily. Vessels in the forearm of toddlers are obscured by cutaneous tissue as well. The scalp veins in the younger child are visible and dilate easily but they are hard to stabilize. Other sites include umbilical cord use or location into either the superior or inferior vena cava.

UNIQUE CATHETER INSERTION TECHNIQUES WITH PEDIATRIC PATIENTS

In order to insert a catheter in a child, often veins are located using moist heat or a **fiber optic transilluminator**. To keep the skin intact, gentle pressure instead of a tourniquet might be used, and tape and alcohol should be used rarely or not at all. Tincture of iodine can affect the thyroid and should be used sparingly. If the scalp vein is used, the catheter should be pointed downward toward the heart. Extremities should be secured including an IV board if necessary. Thermal stability needs to be maintained, especially for the neonate. An environment outside the child's room is preferable. Changing of the catheter should be minimized unless there is a complication, and dressings should be changed at least once a week.

PAIN MANAGEMENT INTERVENTIONS FOR PEDIATRIC PATIENTS

Even though a child cannot communicate as well as an adult, changes in heart rate, oxygen consumption, behavior, or exposure to **situations generally associated with pain require intervention**. Sometimes this intervention can include behavioral support. If a pharmacologic intercession is indicated, some of the types include opioids, local or injectable anesthetics, and transdermal analgesic creams. Local anesthetics are rarely used but injectable ones are typically lidocaine in its hydrochloride or buffered form. Opioids would only be utilized for moderate, severe or chronic pain. The transdermal analgesic creams in current use contain lidocaine as well, either EMLA, which is a mixture of lidocaine-prilocaine anesthetic with a low freezing point, or ELA Max, a 4% topical lidocaine cream. Iontophoresis, a method using an external current to administer the drug into the skin, may be used.

CALCULATING PEDIATRIC MEDICATION DOSAGES

The best way to **calculate pediatric medication dosages** is by use of a nomogram, which is a chart that extrapolates body surface area (BSA) in square millimeters (m^2) based on body weight in kilograms or sometimes pounds. Birth weight should be used for neonates up to one week old. Doses are usually recommended in terms of mg/kg or ug/kg or for chemotherapy in terms of mg/m^2. Therefore, a typical calculation for dosage of a child relative to an adult would be:

Child's dose = (child's BSA in m^2/average adult BSA in m^2) x (adult dose in mg) = mg

Average adult assumptions are for a body surface area of 1.73 m^2. If the dose has been ordered as mg/kg body weight, simple calculation of the dose in mg/kg times the weight in kg might be used as is usually done for adults.

CALCULATING FLUID REQUIREMENTS FOR CHILDREN

There are several ways to **calculate the maintenance fluid requirements for children.** Various formulas are based on the child's weight in kilograms, their body surface area (BSA) in square meters, or their metabolic rate. For children that weigh more than 10 kg, there are standard nomogram charts available that extrapolate the BSA on a plot from the weight and height

40

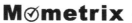

measurements; normally, 1200 to 1500 mL/m² should be infused per day. Another guideline is that 1 mL of water is needed for every calorie consumed; caloric consumption is greatest for weights between 10 and 20 kg. There are also some guidelines based primarily on the child's weight, which use requirements based on the child's weight in kilograms and divide that by 24 hours to determine the infusion rate in mL/hr. Fluid requirements can increase with increases in temperature, stress, burns, or surgical procedures.

ALTERNATIVE FORMULAS FOR CALCULATING PEDIATRIC MEDICATION DOSAGES

Some alternative formulas for calculating pediatric medication dosages make assumptions about relating a child's age to weight to so-called "average" adults. In each case the adult dose is multiplied by a fraction obtained as follows. The first is Fried's Rule, which is used for an infant under 1 year of age, where the infant's age in months is divided by 150 months. For children 2 years or older, 2 different calculations might be used as alternatives:

- **Clark's Rule**, which divides the child's weight in pounds by the average adult weight of 150 lbs.
- **Young's Rule**, which determines the fraction of the adult dose based on age only as: (child's age in years)/ (child's age in years + 12 years).

ADMINISTRATION OF PEDIATRIC MEDICATIONS

There are several ways to **administer medications to a child**, but the preferred method (also the most accurate) is to use a syringe pump. A syringe is attached to low volume tubing connected near the patient. The syringe is primed and drugs infused continuously at an indicated rate. Sometimes, a child is just given a direct intravenous push of a drug bolus. The buret method employs an in-line calibrated chamber and is typically used for older pediatric patients. The retrograde method utilizes tubing with stopcocks on each end. This tubing is attached to the primary administration set and then primed backwards up into an empty distally placed syringe.

SPECIAL CONSIDERATIONS

A child is growing rapidly with dynamic changes in organ maturity as well. The age, body weight and body surface area of the child are all important parameters. The effectiveness of the drug is greatly affected by the absorption rate, which varies quite a bit with the child's age and the distribution of the drug as a function of percent body water and body surface area. Neonates have a greatly diminished capacity to bind protein, they metabolize the drugs more slowly than adults, and their renal function is diminished. Their body weight can fluctuate greatly requiring dosage recalculation.

Care should be given to providing a latex-free environment during intravenous administration to a pediatric patient. In addition, the possibility of exposing the patient to Di(2-ethylhexyl) phthalate, or DEHP, should be avoided because DEHP can leach into the solutions. This can be aided by using polyvinyl chloride devices that do not contain DEHP; the list of devices includes IV bags, administration sets, umbilical catheters and the like. Use plastic solution containers, controlled volume administration sets, and Luer-Loc connections to secure each connection if possible.

DEHYDRATION

The most common type of **dehydration** is **isotonic dehydration** (70%), which means that water and electrolytes are somehow lost at about the same rate from both the intra- and extracellular fluid compartments. Isotonic dehydration usually emanates from gastroenteritis resulting in severe diarrhea, although other causes include fever, vomiting, hemorrhage, burns, excessive urination, or suppression of fluid intake. If a child has isotonic dehydration, they present with thirst, drastic weight loss, dry mucous membranes, cold extremities, a minimal but rapid pulse and a variety of other signs. Sometimes rehydration by mouth is sufficient but otherwise replacement therapy should be instituted.

HYPERTONIC DEHYDRATION

Hypertonic dehydration, sometimes called hypernatremic dehydration, refers to the condition that develops when more water is lost than electrolytes or excessive amounts of the solute are taken in. There are several situations where this often occurs. Some children with diarrhea lose more water than electrolytes. Neonates and infants are often fed high-solute replacement fluids or concentrated formulas and hypertonic dehydration results without proper monitoring. In small infants, fever with rapid breathing can produce this condition. Both types of diabetes can result in hypertonic dehydration, either through movement of water out of the cells into the ECF (mellitus type) or lack of antidiuretic hormone (insipidus type). Symptoms include loose stools, increased thirst, altered electrolyte levels, central nervous system effects, rigidity, weight loss, and others. Bleeding with the brain can actually occur in some infants with this condition. Slow replacement over about a 2-day with a dilute sodium solution in 5% dextrose is generally indicated.

PYLORIC STENOSIS

Pyloric stenosis is a condition in which the circular muscle of the pylorus, which is the opening between the stomach and bowel, becomes hypertrophied or enlarged. The gastric outlet becomes obstructed and distention and vomiting generally result. The condition is much more prevalent with male neonates than females. The exact mechanism is not known but the origins seem to be genetic. Initially, the neonate is just extremely hungry and somewhat dehydrated and malnourished but eventually they develop an observable pyloric mass, massive vomiting, metabolic alkalosis, and other symptoms of dehydration and hyponatremia. The child should be given only intravenous fluids including glucose, and ultimately, they usually need to undergo a surgical procedure called pyloromyotomy, which relieves the obstruction.

HEMOLYTIC DISEASE OF THE NEWBORN

Hemolytic Disease of the Newborn can result from two different types of reactions between antibodies of the mother and the child.

- The most common type results from an **ABO incompatibility** where the mother is O blood group or some variation where she has either anti-A or anti-B antibodies or both which cross the placenta into the type A, B, or AB fetus. Thus, there is an antigen-antibody reaction resulting in the hemolysis of the red blood cells of the fetus. Fetal symptoms include jaundice, anemia, hepatosplenomegaly, and high levels of unconjugated bilirubin, which usually resolve with either phototherapy or only one RBC transfusion.
- A similar hemolytic response can occur in the fetus if an **Rh-negative** mother develops anti-Rh antibodies to her Rh-positive child's antigens and the antibodies are transferred across the placenta. This is also called isoimmunization and symptoms are usually more severe including a condition called erythroblastosis fetalis where undifferentiated red blood cells are found in the circulation of the fetus. Treatments include intramuscular administration of maternal RhoGAM antibodies to prevent problems in future pregnancies, phototherapy, or exchange transfusions in the newborn.

HYPOGLYCEMIA IN INFANTS

In an infant, a blood glucose level of less than 40 to 45 mg/dL indicates **hypoglycemia**, which occurs as a result of either inadequate glucose or dextrose nutrition, too much production of insulin, or high glucose needs accompanying illness. The infant would be jittery, lethargic, limp,

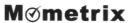

irritable, confused, and would lack the energy to feed themselves orally. Severe hypoglycemia can lead to convulsions or seizures, increased epinephrine secretion and associated side effects, low body temperature, and breathing and heart complications. The infant should be infused through either a large peripheral or central vein with high concentrations of dextrose as well given oral glucose.

SALICYLATE INTOXICATION

Salicylate intoxication, or salicylism, results from toxic levels of salicylate in the serum. It is defined as a serum salicylate level of greater than 150mg/kg. For an infant, this condition can develop if the mother has ingested toxic quantities of salicylate as aspirin or one of its formulations, or topical formulations such as oil of wintergreen have been applied. Decreased gastric mobility occurs causing gastrointestinal problems. Metabolic changes ensue, as well as respiratory problems, dehydration as a result of hyperventilation, and abnormal neurologic, kidney, liver, blood, and diaphoretic functions develop. In order to prevent further absorption of the salicylate, gastric lavage is performed or vomiting is induced. If acetaminophen was present, its antidote N-acetylcysteine would be given. Isotonic solutions are administered to establish adequate blood volume and other electrolytes or supplements given as needed.

CYSTIC FIBROSIS

Cystic fibrosis is a condition that is inherited as an autosomal recessive trait, particularly in Caucasians. In patients with this condition, there is an abnormal secretion of sweat and saliva which results in extremely thick mucus. These individuals are prone to infection because bacteria adhere to the mucous. As this mucous forms precipitates or it coagulates, it begins to obstruct the pancreas and bronchioles and other organs eventually become involved. There is a high concentration of sodium and chloride in the sweat, which means more salt intake is required. Progressive chronic obstructive pulmonary disease develops along with concurrent side effects. In a small percentage of newborns with cystic fibrosis, the intestine becomes blocked, and other gastrointestinal disorders continue throughout the patient's life as a result of the thick intestinal secretions. Treatments range the gamut as needed from chest physiotherapy to IV or oral antibiotics, pancreatic enzyme replacement, nutrition or electrolyte replacement, and even lung transplantation or gene therapy.

MENINGITIS IN INFANTS

Typically, a child of up to 5 years of age is the most susceptible to **meningitis**, which is a condition where the membranes surrounding the brain and spinal cord (meninges) and the underlying subarachnoid space and cerebrospinal fluid become inflamed, white blood cells accumulate and tissue damage occurs. Both bacterial and viral agents are known to cause meningitis, including *Haemophilus influenzae, Streptococcus pneumoniae, Neisseria meningitides,* and tuberculin bacilli. The agent is usually spread through the nasopharynx to underlying vessels and then the blood supply to the brain, but it can be introduced through some type of wound or puncture. Clinical manifestations are numerous including sensorium alterations. Some are organism specific. Neonates develop jaundice, poor or high-pitched cry and poor appetite. The bacterial forms of meningitis constitute a medical emergency including infection control and isolation procedures, and the patient is given acetaminophen and IV antibiotics. Intracranial pressure needs to be reduced hydration maintained, and anemia reversed through blood administration.

> **Review Video: <u>Meningitis</u>**
> Visit mometrix.com/academy and enter code: 277418

43

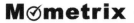

SICKLE CELL ANEMIA

Sickle cell anemia is a disease that is inherited as an autosomal-recessive gene, primarily by blacks and some whites of Mediterranean heritage. With this condition, the individuals possess an abnormal hemoglobin, termed HbS, which results in a crescent or sickle-shaped red blood cell. Clinical manifestations occur only after the fetal hemoglobin disappears. These sickle-shaped RBCs obstruct the smaller blood vessels, the spleen becomes infiltrated and enlarged by these cells putting the patient at risk for infection, and eventually a myriad of other effects can occur. The latter can include liver failure, necrosis and cirrhosis, anemia and inadequate blood supply to the kidneys and bones. Stroke or other brain-related complications are prevalent. Blood transfusions, antibiotics, oxygen therapy and bone marrow transplantation are just a sampling of the extreme measures these individuals might need to control this disease as well as preventive measures such as avoiding sources of infection and rougher sports.

NECROTIZING ENTEROCOLITIS

Necrotizing enterocolitis is an acute inflammatory bowel disease that occurs primarily in premature infants or sometimes other neonates. Its exact cause is unknown but it generally occurs when the gastrointestinal tract of the neonate has been suppressed and it stops producing lubricating mucous permitting enzymes to attack the intestinal wall. Use of hypertonic formulas or medications sometimes exacerbates this condition. A hallmark of this condition is a distended abdomen, but laboratory results usually reveal other findings including blood cell abnormalities, metabolic acidosis, electrolyte imbalances, and sometimes thrombocytopenia. No oral feedings should be given. In extreme cases, the bowel may become perforated which indicates surgical correction by resection and rejoining or creation of an artificial opening.

AIDS IN INFANTS

The **Human Immunodeficiency Virus type I (HIV-I)** can be perinatally acquired by a child while in the uterus or through breast feeding and ultimately, they develop **Acquired Immunodeficiency Syndrome, or AIDS.** In other instances, AIDS can be transmitted via sexual contact or through blood exposure. A decreased number of what are known as CD4 T-cells exists (less than 200 cells/mcL), and B-cell function is depressed as well. If the child was infected by the mother, symptoms usually appear by the time they are about a year and a half old. These clinical manifestations include repeated bacterial infections, lymphadenopathy, hepatosplenomegaly, some cancers such as Kaposi's sarcoma, repeated pulmonary diseases, chronic diarrhea, recurring candidiasis, and neurological problems. Current treatments target slowing the progression of the virus, replacing B cell functions with IV gamma globulin, antibiotic therapy for pneumonia, and nutritional adjuncts.

HEMOPHILIA

The term **hemophilia** refers to an inherited blood disorder in which one of the factors required for blood coagulation is either absent or malfunctioning. Coagulation is therefore suppressed and the patient often bleeds. Classic hemophilia or hemophilia A is a deficit in factor VIII and is the most prevalent, about three-fourths of cases. There are two other types, Hemophilia B or Christmas disease where factor IX, plasma thromboplastin component is deficient, and Hemophilia C where factor XI, a precursor to plasma-thromboplastin, is lacking. In any case, they are all transmitted as X-linked recessive alleles or precipitated by gene mutations. The tendency to bleed can range from moderate to severe depending on how much the factor is depressed. Young children with hemophilia are usually treated by infusing the missing factor several times a week at home after instruction to the parents. A vascular access device is usually implanted. There are some drug therapies available too including desmopressin acetate to release factor VIII and the antifibrinolytic drug Amicar.

LEUKEMIA

Leukemia is a malignant disorder involving an unrestrained rapid increase in the number of immature white blood cells in the bone marrow, spleen and lymphatic tissue. There are two forms found in children, acute lymphocytic leukemia and acute myelocytic leukemia, and they present similarly. The causes of leukemia are not known, but it may have some genetic component and often occurs after some disruption such as exposure to radiation, infection, or chemicals. Clinically, the patient has anemia and is fatigued, they may have fever or infection, bone or joint pain, weight loss, abdominal pain, heightened intracranial pressure, tachycardia and shortness of breath. A catheter is usually inserted into a central vein for vascular access functions. Treatment measures can include chemotherapy at high levels, bone marrow transplantation, and whole-body irradiation.

COMMON CHILDHOOD MALIGNANCIES

Wilms' tumor is a solitary tumor that originates from the renoblast cells of the kidney. Larger Wilms' tumors can cross the midline and obstruct the inferior vena cava or possibly the intestines. This tumor usually grows very fast and metastasizes into the lungs and liver. Surgical intervention is generally removal of the infected kidney. A **neuroblastoma** is a soft but dense tumor that begins in the neural crest cells, which are the progenitors to the adrenal medulla and sympathetic nervous system. Therefore, a neuroblastoma can occur in any area with sympathetic nerve tissue, but it is usually found in the abdominal area, the adrenal gland or the paraspinal ganglia. It is the most common solid tumor located outside the brain presenting in children and the most common malignancy in infants. In addition to surgical resection, chemotherapy, radiation, bone marrow transplantation or immunotherapy might be advised.

BILIARY ATRESIA

Fibrosis of extrahepatic ducts can lead to the blockage of bile flow, known as **biliary atresia**. Bile cannot enter the duodenum so it is stored in the ducts and the gallbladder, which leads to impairment of digestion and fat absorption, biliary cirrhosis and possibly death. Symptoms of this abnormality subtly appear starting with jaundice at about 1 week and proceeding to greenish brown skin (from an uptick in bilirubin), to change in stool color, dark urine, liver cirrhosis, portal hypertension, bleeding and anemia. If left untreated, the patient usually dies during the first few years of life. A hepatic portoenterostomy, which dissects and resects the bile duct, should be done shortly after birth for a good prognosis. A liver transplant can be attempted as well.

COGNITIVE FUNCTION CHANGES AS ADULTS AGE

Cognitive changes related to age vary among individuals but are usually not evident until >70. Studies have shown that by age 81, about 60-70% of people have a small decline in cognitive abilities. *Fluid intelligence* (information processing skills) tends to decline slightly with age while *crystallized intelligence* (acquired knowledge and applied problem solving) is more likely to stay intact or improve. Older adults may have more difficulty in completing complex tasks that require processing of new information. They may become more easily distracted and less able to focus attention. Processing information and reacting may be slowed so that those >60 require more time to complete mental tasks even though their intellectual capability remains intact. Working memory declines making it more difficult for older adults to complete mental processes that require keeping facts in memory (such as calculating costs and tips). Implicit memories (skills, reactions) usually remain intact while explicit memories (facts, information) may decline. Older adults often have difficulty retrieving words (names of people or objects). A steady decline in memory or periods of confusion require further examination.

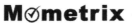

ISSUES AFFECTING OLDER ADULTS
NUTRITIONAL STATUS

A number of changes that occur in older adults may impact **nutritional status**, and many medications may exacerbate these changes:

- Decreased lean body mass and metabolic rate (decreases 2% each decade).
- Decreased production of saliva and gastric acids.
- Decreased bone mineralization.
- Decreased perception of thirst, decreased sense of smell and taste.
- Increased cholecystokinin, leading to early feeling of satiety.

While older adults are often less active than younger adults and require fewer calories, they still require the same vitamins and minerals and may, in fact, require more. For each decade over age 30, males usually need 7 fewer calories and females 10 fewer. Conditions, such as anorexia, dysphagia, constipation, and malnutrition are common in older adults. Older adults who live/eat alone often fail to prepare adequate meals, and decreased income may prevent people from buying nutritious foods. Loss of teeth may limit food choices.

DRUG DOSES AND CALCULATIONS

Older adults often take 4 to 5 different **drugs**, increasing the risk of polypharmacy, drug interactions, and adverse effects. Because of alterations in rates of absorption (often decreased but sometimes increased), dosages should start low, often at one-third to one-half of a standard dose and then be titrated slowly upward if needed. Some medications (those listed as part of the Beers criteria) should be avoided or given at very low doses to older adults because of frequent adverse effects. Patients must be monitored carefully and kidney and liver function assessed at least annually with laboratory tests because liver or renal disease may impact pharmacokinetics. Additionally, changes associated with aging may affect all phases of pharmacokinetics:

- **Absorption**: Gastric pH is les acidic, villi are decreased, and motility slows.
- **Distribution**: Water content decreases, fat content increases, and protein binding sites are reduced.
- **Metabolism**: Hepatic metabolism slows.
- **Excretion**: Neurons decrease, GFR decreases up to 50%.

GERONTOLOGICAL DISEASES/CONDITIONS THAT MAY REQUIRE INFUSION THERAPY
CONGESTIVE HEART FAILURE

Congestive heart failure is a cardiac disease that includes disorders of contractions (systolic dysfunction) or filling (diastolic dysfunction) or both and may include pulmonary, peripheral, or systemic edema. Congestive heart failure is an end-stage of heart failure in which edema is pronounced. With congestive heart failure, systolic heart failure (typical left-sided) tends to occur first followed by diastolic (right-sided). Over time, the heart muscle begins to lose contractibility and blood begins to pool in the ventricles during contractions, stretching the myocardium and enlarging the ventricles. The heart compensates by thickening the muscle without an adequate increase in capillary blood supply because of the vasoconstriction of the coronary arteries, leading to ischemia. Ejection fractions decrease, resulting in decreased cardiac output. The most common causes are coronary artery disease, systemic or pulmonary hypertension, cardiomyopathy, and valvular disorders. The incidence of chronic heart failure correlates with age. Medications may include ACE inhibitors, ARBs, BBs, CCBs, and other vasodilators. For advanced disease, IV medications, such as dobutamine and/or milrinone, may be administered to improve pumping action and diuretics, such as furosemide, to reduce edema.

SEVERE DEHYDRATION

Older adults conserve water less effectively, have a less-pronounced sense of thirst, and may have impaired sodium balance. Lean body mass decreases from 65% to 40% replaced by increased fat and decreases total body water. **Dehydration** occurs when total body water decreases but total body sodium does not, resulting from inadequate fluid intake, excess water loss, especially in hot weather, disease nasogastric suctioning, drugs, diarrhea, vomiting, and fever:

- **Mild**: (5% loss) Dizziness, lethargy, altered mentation, reduced skin turgor, and dry mucous membranes, orthostatic hypotension.
- **Moderate**: (10% loss) Confusion, resting hypotension, tachycardia, and oliguria/anuria.
- **Severe**: (>15%) Marked hypotension and anuria in addition to other symptoms.

Diagnosis includes increased hematocrit, BUN/creatinine ratio, and Na (>20 mEq/L). *Treatment* includes estimating fluid loss and replacing 50% in the first 12 hours:

- **Mild to moderate**: Increase oral fluids (2-3 liters) or IV fluids (0.9% NS).
- **Severe**: IV fluid intake should be adequate to resolve orthostatic hypotension and cardiac dysrhythmias within 24 hours, and then the remaining fluid loss can be replaced more slowly.

OSTEOPOROSIS

Osteoporosis is characterized by thin porous bones that break easily because of low bone mass and structural deterioration, with more bone lost than gained. Osteoporosis is most common in post-menopausal women although men >65 lose bone at the same rate as women. Primary osteoporosis is part of normal aging. Bone mass density (BMD) testing can identify the extent of osteoporosis. A history of older adults should include assessment of risk factors:

F	Fractures
R	Race
A	Age and gender
C	Chronic disease/ medications
T	Thin bones, low weight
U	Underactive: inadequate exercise
R	Reduced estrogen
E	Excessive alcohol intake & smoking
D	Diet

Cancer survivors and those with chronic diseases are often at increased risk because of metabolic changes and/or medications, such as corticosteroids. Treatments include oral bisphosphonates, selective estrogen receptor modulator, calcitonin, and recombinant human parathyroid hormone.

Other treatments include diets rich in calcium and vitamin D, balance training, strength training, and regular weight-bearing exercise. Two bisphosphonates are given by intravenous infusion:

- Ibandronate (Boniva®): Administered quarterly.
- Zoledronic acid (Reclast®: Administered annually.

> **Review Video: Osteoporosis**
> Visit mometrix.com/academy and enter code: 421205

ANEMIA

Anemia results in a decrease in oxygen transportation and decreased perfusion throughout the body, causing the heart to compensate by increasing cardiac output. As the blood becomes less viscous, there is decreased peripheral resistance, so more blood is pumped to the heart, and this increased flow can cause turbulence that results in a heart murmur and, if severe or prolonged, heart failure. Anemia is commonly caused by hemorrhage, hemolysis, hematopoiesis, or lack of adequate dietary iron.

Symptoms include:

- General malaise and weakness.
- Poor feeding/ anorexia.
- Pallor.
- Shortness of breath on exertion.
- Headache, dizziness.
- Apathy, depression, decreased attention span, slowed thought processes.
- Shock symptoms (with severe blood loss):
  o Tachycardia
  o Hypotension
  o poor peripheral circulation
  o pallor

Treatment:

- Identification and treatment of underlying cause.
- Blood or blood components as indicated.
- Supportive care: oxygen, intravenous fluids.
- Splenectomy (for hemolytic anemias).
- Oral or IV iron (for iron deficiency).

IMPACT OF PREGNANCY ON FLUID AND NUTRITIONAL STATUS

During pregnancy, the **nutrition** of the mother has a profound effect on the developing embryo/fetus. Caloric needs vary widely depending on the mother's age, size, weight, metabolism, and general health. Energy needs of the mother usually remain stable during the first trimester, but an additional **300 kilocalories** a day are needed during the second and third trimesters for a singleton, and **600 kilocalories** a day for twins. Recommended nutrient intake for pregnant women is shown below:

Vit. A (μg/d)	Vit. C (mg/d)	Vit. D (μg/d)	Vit. E (mg/d)	Vit. K (μg/d)	Ca (mg/d)	Phos. (mg/d)
750- 770	80-85	≥5	15	75-90	1000-1300	700-1250

48

Generally, a pregnant woman requires about 71 g of **protein** daily (3 meat servings or equivalent) and 4 to 5 cups of milk (or equivalent). Diet should include 2 to 4 servings of fruit and 3 to 5 servings of vegetables. **Simple carbohydrates** (sugar, flour) should be limited and replaced by whole grains, which are high in B vitamins. **Fat** should constitute about 30% of total caloric intake. Iron intake should be about 27mg per day.

CONSIDERATIONS WHEN INFUSING PREGNANT PATIENTS

When administering an **infusion to a pregnant patient**, the risks to both the patient and the fetus must be considered. Issues to consider include:

- **FDA classification of drug:** A category means well-controlled studies have demonstrated no adverse effect. B category means animal studies show no adverse effect but well-controlled studies have not been carried out on pregnant women OR animal studies show adverse effects but studies on pregnant women do not. C category is inconclusive, and D and X demonstrate danger to the fetus.
- **Dosage calculated per kg/body weight:** Base dosage on current pregnant weight.
- **Hydration status:** Fluids should achieve euvolemia, so fluid excess should be avoided. With hyperemesis gravidarum, the patient may be severely dehydrated. If rehydrating the patient, thiamine should be administered before IV fluids containing glucose because of increased risk of Wernicke encephalopathy.
- **Presence of labor:** Fluids are usually administered before an epidural.

INFUSION THERAPY FOR INDIVIDUALS WITH CHRONIC RENAL CONDITIONS

When considering **infusion therapy in patients with chronic renal disease** it is important to understand the impact that this disease has on the body's ability to filter and excrete drugs. When kidneys are damaged, filtration and excretion decrease, so flow rates and dosages must be adapted to accommodate these changes. Otherwise, medications can accumulate into possibly lethal amounts.

Infusion therapy has also proven effective in the **treatment and management** of the symptoms of chronic renal disease, as well as following kidney transplant. The following infusion therapies are most common in patients suffering from chronic renal disease:

- **Iron**: Iron deficiency anemia is common in patients with chronic renal disease that are receiving dialysis, but can also occur in CKD patients that are not dependent on dialysis.
- **Rituximab**: Given to reduce B-cells that cause immune related kidney disease caused by vasculitis.
- **Magnesium**: Given to replace magnesium in patients deficient of this electrolyte due to the kidney's inability to regulate magnesium absorption.
- **IVIG:** Given post-kidney transplant to reduce the risk of organ rejection.

Infusion Therapies

Infusion Therapy Initiation and Monitoring

INITIATING INFUSION THERAPY

Infusion is usually initiated for therapeutic reasons but sometimes it is done for diagnostic purposes. When a patient cannot sustain adequate intake independently, therapeutic infusion is started to maintain levels of water, electrolytes, nutrients, or nitrogen or to reequilibrate the acid-base balance. Medications, whole blood or its components, anesthetics, or pain relievers, if needed, constitute the main reasons to begin infusions. Infusion may also be started in order to administer some type of diagnostic reagent or to monitor hemodynamic function. In emergency situations, infusion is sometimes begun just to maintain unblocked vascular access.

PATIENT ASSESSMENT NECESSARY BEFORE INITIATING INFUSION THERAPY

Prior to administering infusion therapy, the health care professional must be armed with a variety of information. Some of this information is knowledge of the patient's history, including primary and secondary diagnoses, conditions responsive to the therapy, possible side effects or allergies, and prior history of respiratory or coagulation issues, previous transfusions or fluid/electrolyte imbalances. A variety of laboratory data should be obtained prior to therapy. In particular, evaluations of renal function such as blood urine nitrogen (BUN); electrolyte levels; complete blood count (CBC) and percentages of its components; coagulation issues such as platelet levels and prothrombin time; and respiratory state if needed determined by drawing arterial blood gases. Physical assessment of the patient should be done including vital signs, fluid taken in and excreted, skin and tongue turgor, observations of fluid volume deficit, presence of swelling, and changes in body weight.

HISTORY QUESTIONS OR CLINICAL INDICATORS TO ASSESS BEFORE DRUG ADMINISTRATION

Before giving a patient any drugs, the nurse or other provider should question the individual about their **historical health status, presence of any allergies and use of medications.** Clinically, basic data like age, weight, height, and body temperature should be known prior to drug administration. The skin should be examined for its elastic properties and appearance including the presence of any rashes or wounds or redness. Any swelling or other means of fluid loss such as vomiting or diarrhea should be documented. The patient should be observed for their ability to respond to sensory stimulation.

LABORATORY TESTING WHEN MEDICATING PATIENTS

A number of **clinical chemistry and hematology tests** should be performed for patients being given drugs:

- **Blood tests** include coagulation parameters, chemical analysis of components, and cell counts.
- A **urine sample** is typically taken to analyze its properties often including the pattern of drug elimination.
- **Therapeutic drug monitoring** may be done in which test samples are taken at intervals after administering a single drug dose and then measuring the time to maximum and minimum drug concentrations present in the blood.
- Other screening tests could include bacterial sensitivity or resistance or toxicology screens.

50

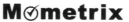

INFORMATION DOCUMENTED EVERY TIME A DRUG IS ADMINISTERED

For legal purposes to protect themselves, when giving drugs the nurse should **document** all of the following information:

- Drug administered.
- Dose given.
- Rate administered.
- Time period given.
- Route of administration.
- Response by the patient to the medication.

Additional documentation is required for high-risk infusions, particularly blood products. While this is specific to hospital policy, generally blood transfusions require vitals be taken prior to administration initiation, 5 minutes after initiation, and specific time increments thereafter. This is meant to ensure early detection of dangerous reactions to blood transfusions.

Legally, each individual (in this case the nurse) is liable for their own actions and could be held accountable. Offenses could include negligence, battery or untoward bodily touching, and assault (fear of impending bodily harm). In the hospital, protocols are usually established by the Institutional Review Board. In non-hospital settings such as infusion centers, clinics, or doctors' offices the same standards apply.

ADMIXING

Admixing is the process by which medications are prepared or compounded. It is usually performed by the pharmacy in a clean, assigned area usually under a laminar flow hood. The hood greatly eliminates the possibility of including bacteria or other microorganisms from the air, especially if good sterile technique is used. Admixing should only be performed after considering the compatibility of the components in terms of whether untenable chemical or physical changes could occur or whether the drug effectiveness of the medication can be maintained. Parameters to consider include drug concentration, pH, buffering capacity, and the length of contact time with diluents or other components before giving the drug to the patient.

DRESSINGS

Dressings are of two types, either sterile gauze or transparent semipermeable membrane (TSM) dressings. These dressings are aseptically applied after site insertion over the site and replaced whenever they appear damp, loose, or visibly soiled. The edges of gauze dressing should always be taped, but tape may compromise the properties of TSM dressings and interfere with the ability to see the site. When used together, the gauze dressing is usually covered with a TSM dressing. When changing dressings applied to central vascular sites, sterile gloves and a mask should be worn.

INSERTION OF CATHETER INTO VENTRICULAR RESERVOIR

Sometimes a receptacle attached to a catheter is surgically inserted into the **lateral ventricle of the brain** and then connected to the spinal space. By inserting a 25-gauge or smaller needle into this reservoir, two-way access to the brain or cerebrospinal fluid (CSF) is provided. Fluid can be injected or removed and medication can be delivered into the CSF. The need for repeated lumbar punctures is obviated with this technique. The drawbacks to this application are that infection or clogging can occur and strict sterile technique must be employed.

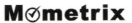

CATHETER REMOVAL

A physician's order is needed to **discontinue infusion therapy** and can depend on a number of factors. The general guidelines are outlined in the *Infusion Nursing Standards of Practice.* For a short peripheral catheter, the health care provider should use good aseptic technique and apply pressure and a dry sterile bandage. Midline peripheral catheters may have had a dwell time as long as 4 weeks, so additional precautions are necessary including immediate removal if contamination or complications are suspected and applying antiseptic ointments. For arterial sites, pressure with the fingers needs to be applied upon removal until hemostasis occurs before applying dressings. When removing peripherally inserted central catheters, it is important to take precautions against development of air embolism. This is also true for central devices that were neither tunneled nor implanted. On the other hand, both tunneled central vascular access devices and implanted central vascular access ports should be removed by a physician, not the nurse.

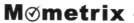

Pain Management

ANALGESIC

An **analgesic** is a drug that is given to alleviate pain without concurrent loss of consciousness. Each has some sort of effect on the central nervous system. Some are actually narcotics and do induce drowsiness or dizziness or blurred vision. Morphine sulfate is one of the most well-known analgesics, used to treat severe pain, but it must be used cautiously because it can cause respiratory or circulatory side effects or allergic reactions. Other analgesics include dezocine (Dalgan), nalbuphine hydrochloride (Nubain), buprenorphine hydrochloride (Buprenex Injection), hydromorphone hydrochloride (Dilaudid), meperidine (Demerol) and fentanyl citrate.

INTRATHECAL ANALGESIA

In **intrathecal analgesia**, a narcotic is delivered directly to the spinal cord. To minimize risk, the catheter is usually inserted between the lumbar vertebrae into the cord, and the dosage and interval of administration greatly reduced relative to that of epidural procedures. Intrathecal analgesia is commonly utilized for patients with chronic pain syndrome or those undergoing simultaneous chemotherapy, antibiotic therapy or anesthesia. The same precautions required for epidural analgesia apply for intrathecal. The medication can be delivered by an implantable pump, an external pump, or a ventricular reservoir.

NARCAN

Narcan, or naloxone hydrochloride, is a drug that structurally resembles morphine. It is used to reverse the effects of morphine sulfate or other analgesics resembling it, like hydromorphone hydrochloride or fentanyl citrate. Narcan should always be readily available when these drugs are administered and given if necessary to treat narcotic-induced depression. Naloxone hydrochloride blocks morphine receptor cells thereby preventing the action of morphine or the other narcotics.

SEDATIVES, HYPNOTICS, OR ANXIOLYTICS

Some drugs affect the central nervous system (CNS) by **sedating, hypnotizing, or relieving the patient's anxiety.** These would be classified as sedatives, hypnotics or anxiolytics. Examples of drugs falling into these categories include diazepam (Valium), lorazepam (Ativan), chlordiazepoxide hydrochloride (Librium), phenobarbital sodium, and bupivacaine hydrochloride (Marcaine). Each has a slightly different indication. Phenobarbital is used to induce lengthy sedation. Lorazepam is usually given before anesthesia to prevent vomiting. Marcaine is used for pain control. Valium and Librium are really anxiolytics because they are used to treat psychoneurotic or critical stress reactions, trembling, or alcohol withdrawal. Another CNS agent, fosphenytoin sodium (Cerebyx), acts to stop convulsions.

EPIDURAL ANESTHESIA

During **epidural anesthesia**, a physician inserts a catheter into the epidural space in the lumbar region of the spinal cord. Then either the physician or nurse administers medications, which can be of low, intermediate, or high strength and different times of action. The anesthetics diffuse through the relatively thin dura and arachnoid membranes to spread. This is useful during many surgeries because sensory and motor responses in the lower half of the body are blocked. The procedure is also used in obstetrics. In either case, heart rates, respiratory status, arterial pressure, or electrocardiogram pattern should be closely monitored.

EPIDURAL ANALGESIA

Epidural analgesia is typically performed in cases of acute pain after surgery or for chronic pain syndrome, whereas epidural anesthesia is given before some surgeries. The analgesic medication dulls the sensory response to pain without loss of consciousness. Medications do not contain preservatives and are continuously administered by an electronic diffusion device through a 0.2-micron filter devoid of surfactant. Examples include morphine, methadone, hydromorphone, and fentanyl. The more lipid-soluble the drug is, the faster it acts because it can diffuse across a lipid membrane to relieve pain. As these agents are narcotics, Narcan must be available as an antidote and the patient must be observed for systemic complications.

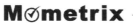

Cardiovascular Infusions

AGENTS FOR HYPOTENSION

The most commonly used drugs for **hypotension** are dopamine hydrochloride (Intropin) and norepinephrine bitartrate (Levophed). Both are given continuously with an electronic infusion device starting with low doses and then increasing or adjusting the dosage to maintain optimal blood pressure. Cardiac side effects and possible tissue damage if the agents leak can occur. The nurse must monitor blood pressure every few minutes. The health care provider should also be ready to administer an antidote if necessary; the antidote of choice is injection of phentolamine mesylate (Regitine) diluted into 0.9% saline. In acute emergency hypotensive situations, another drug called metaraminol bitartrate (Aramine) might be injected.

DRUGS FOR HYPERTENSION

Drugs available to treat **hypertension** include labetalol hydrochloride (Normodyne), methyldopa hydrochloride (Aldomet), nitroprusside sodium (Nipride), nitroglycerin (Tridil), and hydralazine hydrochloride (Apresoline). Nipride and Apresoline are also utilized to treat shock to the cardiac system, the latter actually being a vasodilator. Nitroglycerin is used to treat hypertension during surgery and it is also used to relieve congestive heart failure concomitant with acute myocardial infarction. If a patient is experiencing an acute hypertensive crisis, the drug of choice might be either Aldomet or Nipride.

AGENTS USED FOR TACHYCARDIA

Tachycardia, or rapid heartbeat, can be treated by a number of drugs. The drug of choice may be selected based on the type of tachycardia, and some of these agents have antiarrhythmic properties as well.

- **Bretylium tosylate, or Bretylate,** is generally indicated for treatment of unresponsive rapid heartbeats in the ventricle.
- **Esmolol hydrochloride, or Brevibloc,** is usually administered if a patient has supraventricular tachycardia, which is characterized as a very fast pulse above 140 beats per minute.
- **Propranolol hydrochloride, or Inderal,** is normally given to treat sudden rapid beats in the atrium or sinus areas, or atrial flutter and fibrillation.
- When lidocaine cannot be used, a drug called **procainamide hydrochloride, or Pronestyl,** might be administered to treat tachycardia; however, this agent can cause a drug-induced systemic lupus syndrome.

DRUGS FOR CARDIAC ARRHYTHMIAS

Arrhythmia is an irregular heartbeat or rhythm. The most common drugs utilized to treat cardiac arrhythmia include digoxin (Lanoxin), lidocaine hydrochloride (Xylocaine), verapamil hydrochloride (Isoptin), and quinidine gluconate. Digoxin actually has a wide range of applications, including not only treatment of abnormal heartbeat patterns in the ventricle accompanying congestive heart failure, but also problems in the atrium and cardiogenic shock. Digitalis toxicity must be monitored. Irregular heartbeats originating at or near the ventricle might be treated with xylocaine or Isoptin. Adenosine (Adenocard), a vasodilator, might be given when there is an abnormal sinus rhythm.

TREATMENT IF PATIENT'S HEART STOPS

If a patient has an **atrioventricular heart block and their heart stops**, they are normally given isoproterenol hydrochloride, or Isuprel Hydrochloride. This is administered either by push or

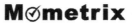

continuously using an electronic infusion control device. The patient should be instructed to report any chest pain or other side effects to the health care provider. Chest pain, or angina, can be caused by lack of blood to the heart. Palpitations, sweating, facial flush and gastrointestinal problems might be further side effects.

EPINEPHRINE HYDROCHLORIDE

Epinephrine hydrochloride (Adrenalin chloride) is the drug of first defense to treat anaphylactic shock or any type of severe histamine overdose or allergic reaction. It is a hormone that relaxes the airways and constricts the blood vessels and therefore allows the individual in anaphylactic shock to resume breathing normally. Epinephrine is usually administered by push. Blood pressure should be checked by the health care professional at frequent intervals for an hour after administration. The patient's sensory ability and anxiety level should be constantly monitored as well.

ELECTROLYTE AGENTS FOR CONGESTIVE HEART FAILURE

Congestive heart failure refers to a condition where the veins become congested because the heart is not able to pump away the blood returning to it quickly enough. Some agents that equilibrate electrolytes or water currently used to treat this condition include bumetanide (Bumex) and ethacrynate sodium (Edecrin Sodium Intravenous). Serum electrolyte profiles and fluid ingestion and excretion should be monitored when giving these agents.

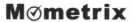

Hematologic Infusions

DRUGS TO TREAT ANEMIA

Anemia is a condition where there are either too few red blood cells or those cells have insufficient hemoglobin. Currently, the drugs available to treat anemia are darbepoetin alfa (Aranesp) and epoetin alfa (EPO, Epogen). Aranesp is usually injected weekly at a dose of 0.45 ug/kg of body weight. EPO or Epogen is usually administered by push; the dosing regimen is dictated by the patient's hematocrit. Both of these drugs can have cardiac side effects and blood pressure should be monitored. Patients should not drive or manage machinery when taking these drugs, and they are usually given a strict dietary regimen.

HEPARIN SODIUM

Heparin sodium is an agent that prevents coagulation by stopping the transformation of prothrombin to thrombin and fibrinogen to fibrin. Therefore, it is usually utilized to prevent or treat thrombosis or blockage of blood vessels by blood clots. Heparin sodium can also prevent the blockage of vascular catheters. Heparin can be administered by push, intermittently, or continuously using an electronic infusion device. The important parameter to check during administration is PTT, or partial thromboplastin time, which should be stabilized at a value greater than and up to 2 times the control. Protamine sulfate negates the effects of heparin sodium and should be available to treat a heparin overdose, which might be indicated by bruises, bleeding gums, or blood in the urine.

> **Review Video: Heparin – An Injectable Anti-Coagulant**
> Visit mometrix.com/academy and enter code: 127426

STREPTOKINASE

Streptokinase, or Streptase, is an enzyme produced by streptococci bacteria. This enzyme dissolves blood clots in humans. Therefore, it is indicated in treatment of pulmonary emboli. Streptokinase is also a plasmin activator and is thus used to treat acute myocardial infarction as well. The doses given to treat severe myocardial infarction are greater than those used to dissolve pulmonary blood clots. Allergic reactions, bleeding or fever can develop with streptokinase administration, and the patient should not use aspirin-containing medications. Another drug, alteplase (Activase), has similar applications.

AMINOCAPROIC ACID OR ANTITHROMBIN III

Aminocaproic acid, available commercially as Amicar Intravenous, is usually given when a patient is actively hemorrhaging as a result of the rapid lysis of fibrin. Cardiac or neurological side effects can occur including grand mal seizure.

Antithrombin III (AT-III, Thrombate III), on the other hand, is a used to routinely treat blood clots. These clots are often pulmonary blood clots so lungs and breathing patterns should be observed. Shortness of breath can be a side effect. The patient should watch for bruises, bleeding gums, blood in the urine, and they should be instructed to avoid aspirin products.

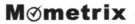

Antineoplastic Infusions

GRANULOCYTE COLONY STIMULATING FACTOR

Granulocyte Colony Stimulating Factor, or G-CSF, is an anti-neutropenic agent. In other words, it is an agent that decreases the time a patient has a low neutrophil or white blood count, or neutropenia. This in turn decreases the likelihood of infection. G-CSF can be administered either in single doses or continuously. This agent is often given to cancer patients, and CBCs and platelet count should be checked before and after chemotherapy begins because an increase in white blood cells, an indication of infection, could occur.

CELL CYCLE

The **cell cycle** is the series of phases that both normal and cancer cells go through. Cells in the body normally divide and enter a resting phase, where they usually remain unless they need to replicate as a result of damage or death. There are **five stages in the cell cycle:**

- G_0: A dormant stage where the cell is not multiplying.
- G_1: Stage where replication is begun through ribonucleic acid (RNA) and protein synthesis.
- **S:** Deoxyribonucleic acid (DNA) is synthesized.
- G_2: The mitotic spindle is manufactured; also called premitosis.
- **M:** Mitosis or actual cells divide and multiply.

EFFECTS ON NORMAL CELL CYCLE WHEN CANCER CELLS DEVELOP

The control mechanism preventing uncontrolled cell division in normal cells is not operating properly in **cancerous cells**. Therefore, the cancer cells keep dividing regardless of need, and they form cell masses or tumors, which can also push into other areas of the body resulting in what is known as metastases. Many cancer cells are actively dividing, some cells may be in a resting phase, and some of the cancer cells are immature. An immature cell is one that is not differentiated into a specific type of cell. The number of cells in a tumor mass is called the tumor burden.

ANTINEOPLASTIC AGENTS

While there are a number of **different types of antineoplastic drugs** now available, the basic purpose of all of them is to prevent cancer cells from dividing by disrupting the cell division process at some point or destroying some component involved in cell division. Many of the agents also have the same effects on normal cells so the key is to either begin therapy early or target the therapy during a time of heavy cell replication. There are two types of antineoplastic agents, ones that are cell cycle-specific and those that are cell cycle-nonspecific:

- The **cell cycle-specific agents** either inhibit or interfere with some part of the cell cycle, and are therefore most effective during heavy replication.
- The **nonspecific agents** target the cells in a resting phase by mechanisms such as chromosomal damage, destruction of DNA, prevention of RNA transcription or other nonselective actions.

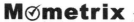

CELL CYCLE-SPECIFIC DRUGS USED IN CANCER TREATMENT

There are two main types of drugs used for cancer treatment that interfere specifically with the cell cycle. The **two main types of cell cycle-specific drugs** used in cancer treatment are either antimetabolites or vinca alkaloids:

- **Antimetabolites** act during the S phase of cell replication by suppressing DNA synthesis and therefore protein synthesis as well. These agents can have some side effects on the blood or gastrointestinal system; they include drugs such as methotrexate, cytarabine, and fluorouracil.
- The **vinca alkaloids** obtained from plants act to prevent cell division during any phase of the cell cycle (except the resting stage) by blocking both DNA and RNA synthesis and binding to the tubules. They can have neurological side effects; these agents include vinblastine, vincristine, and vinorelbine.

CELL CYCLE-NONSPECIFIC AGENTS TO TREAT CANCER

There are a number of types of agents that **act on cells when they are not actively dividing.** These include most alkylating agents, antitumor antibiotics, and nitrosoureas as well as some miscellaneous drugs and biologic agents. The first three types of agents are drugs that interfere in some way with either DNA or RNA:

- **Alkylating agents** such as cisplatin and cyclophosphamide interfere with replication of deoxyribonucleic acid.
- **Antitumor antibiotics** employ several different mechanisms to either interfere with RNA synthesis or to suppress or actually react with DNA. Some examples of antitumor antibiotics include bleomycin, doxorubicin hydrochloride, and mitomycin C.
- **Nitrosoureas** such as carmustine and streptozocin also inhibit DNA replication and repair.

CHEMOTHERAPEUTIC AGENTS WITH STRICT DOSAGE AND LIFETIME CUMULATIVE DOSAGE REQUIREMENTS

The **dosage** of chemotherapeutic agents usually needs to be monitored because of the more severe side effects of bone marrow suppression, cardiotoxicity or other toxicities, or the possibility of a hypersensitivity reaction that could result in anaphylaxis. Some of the antitumor antibiotics have strict dosage and lifetime cumulative dosage requirements. Antibiotics can lose their effectiveness if given in excessive amounts. Drugs that suppress the bone marrow, such as Cerubidine, Adriamycin, or Mutamycin, typically have these strict dosage requirements including lifetime limits.

PLICAMYCIN AS A CHEMOTHERAPEUTIC AGENT

Plicamycin (Mithracin) is generally given to a patient to control the hypercalcemia that accompanies malignant disease by continuous or intermittent infusion. It inhibits bone reabsorption and reduces serum calcium levels. Therefore, in addition to the possible side effects of bone marrow suppression, renal or liver toxicity, and others, actual hypocalcemia might occur if excessive amounts are given. Symptoms might include muscle cramps, weakness, a tingling in the legs or arms, or most importantly facial redness, nosebleeds, and phlebitis. Facial flushing is an early indication of hemorrhage. Be sure to monitor CBCs and electrolyte levels. The health care provider should give no more than a dosage of 25 microgram per kg per day for 3 to 4 days each week to control hypercalcemia. If Mithracin is used to treat testicular cancer, it may be administered for up to 10 days.

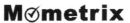

DOXORUBICIN LIPOSOME INJECTION (DOXIL)

Doxorubicin liposome injection (Doxil) had been prepared as a liposome suspension and is therefore an irritant. It is also not compatible with 0.9% saline solutions and must instead be given by intermittent infusion in 5% dextrose in water only. The patient should expect their urine to be red in color for the first few voidings after administration. Doxil may not be well tolerated and in addition to a number of common side effects of chemotherapy it specifically can cause skin or blood side effects. Do not exceed a total cumulative dose of 550 mg/m².

ANTINEOPLASTIC THERAPY

SIDE EFFECTS AND RISKS

Some of the most important **immediate side effects of antineoplastic therapy** include allergic reactions, inflammation of the blood vessels, leaking of fluid from the blood vessels into the surrounding tissues, and gastrointestinal problems. All of these must be closely monitored. Later, a number of **delayed effects** can occur including hair loss (alopecia), suppression of the bone marrow, gastrointestinal problems such as diarrhea, nausea and vomiting, reproductive or sexual issues, changes in ability to taste, increase in mucous, and the possibility of developing psychosocial problems. Toxicity can develop in a number of bodily systems including in the bone marrow, the cardiovascular system, kidneys, the bladder, the liver, the lungs, or the nervous system.

INJECTION SITE REACTIONS

Occasionally antineoplastic agents can cause either **irritation at the site** or actual soft tissue damage. Agents that are possible irritants can cause burning or pain at the site, a buildup of excess fluid, or redness. Some antineoplastic agents are classified as possible vesicants, meaning that they may be actually toxic to soft tissue and cause blistering if the agent leaks into the surrounding tissue. These agents primarily include the group of antitumor antibiotics. If they are to be administered, the infusion site should be closely monitored and if tissue damage is observed or suspected, administration should be stopped.

HEMATOLOGIC COMPLICATIONS WITH CHEMOTHERAPY

The main three types of **hematologic complications** found during chemotherapy administration are neutropenia, thrombocytopenia, and anemia.

- In **neutropenia** there is a decreased white blood cell count with a concurrent decrease in the neutrophil (ANC) count, which predisposes the patient to infection. Therefore, symptoms such as fever and purulent damage and WBC and ANC counts should be monitored, and antibiotics given if infection is confirmed.
- **Thrombocytopenia** is defined as a decrease in platelet count which may result in an increased susceptibility to bleeding. Attention should be paid to bleeding gums or nosebleeds, blood in the urine or stools, easy bruising, or a large spleen or liver. Pressure should be applied to the bleeding and the physician contacted.
- If the oxygen-carrying capacity of the blood is decreased because the number of red blood cells is low, a condition called **anemia** may result. The patient might have a number of cardiac or fatigue-type symptoms. If abnormal hemoglobin or hematocrit is obtained, red blood cells, oxygen, or erythropoietin may be indicated.

GASTROINTESTINAL COMPLICATIONS WITH CHEMOTHERAPY

Common **gastrointestinal complications** of chemotherapy include nausea and vomiting, anorexia, diarrhea, and sometimes constipation. The major risk involved if the first three occur is the possibility of dehydration and insufficient nutritional status. If diarrhea occurs, electrolyte

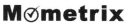

imbalance can also occur. If nausea and vomiting occur, use of antiemetics is usually indicated. If the patient becomes anorexic, high protein or high calorie foods may be prescribed as well as nutritional supplements, appetite stimulants, or even administration of total nutrition parenterally. Serum electrolytes should be monitored, antidiarrheal agents administered, and a high protein, high fluid diet prescribed. Fluid intake also needs to be increased if constipation occurs and a diet high in fiber and bulk prescribed.

CHEMOTHERAPEUTIC AGENTS THAT ADVERSELY AFFECT RENAL FUNCTION

Chemotherapeutic agents that are known to often specifically affect **renal function** including toxicity, hemorrhagic cystitis, and frequent or burning urination. With these drugs, the patient should be given adequate hydration before and after drug administration and they should be encouraged to increase their oral fluid intake and empty their bladder every 4 hours. Laboratory results that should be monitored include BUN, serum creatinine, creatinine clearance, urinalysis and uric acid. The nitrosoureas, which are irritants, often cause renal toxicity, and in the case of streptozocin the urine should be monitored for protein. High dosages of methotrexate, an antimetabolite, often cause renal problems and need to be reversed within 24 hours with leucovorin calcium rescue.

PHASES OF CLINICAL INVESTIGATIONS

Often antineoplastic agents given to cancer patients may actually be administered as part of an investigational protocol. **Clinical investigations** are divided into 4 distinct phases:

- For drugs, **phase I** is designed merely to determine the highest tolerated dose of the drug including toxicities and to examine the pharmacology involved; subjects may be normal individuals.
- **Phase II** for an antitumor drug would involve looking at more defined doses or administration schedules to further evaluate antitumor activity or toxicity.
- In **phase III,** the investigational drug is compared to existing drug protocols, after which the drug can be marketed if the Food and Drug Administration finds favorable results.
- **Phase IV** are trials that give more information about prolonged use of the agent after it has been marketed. In a hospital or other institution where trials are performed, they are internally monitored by the Institutional Review Board.

ALKYLATING AGENTS FOR CANCER TREATMENT

The following are category types and indications for use of **alkylating agents** for cancer treatment:

- **Carboplatin (Paraplatin):** Non-vesicant, indicated for solid tumors such as brain tumors, before bone marrow transplantation, and in a number of other cancers.
- **Cisplatin (Platinol):** An irritant and also a vesicant in high concentration, used to treat neuroblastoma, Wilms' tumor, multiple myeloma, lymphoma, plus other cancers.
- **Cyclophosphamide (Cytoxan):** Non-vesicant, again used to prepare for bone marrow transplantation, and to treat lymphocytic leukemia, Hodgkin's and non-Hodgkin's lymphoma, myeloma, mycosis fungoides, and other tumors.
- **Dacarbazine (DTIC):** Irritant, indicated to treat melanoma, soft tissue sarcomas, neuroblastoma and Hodgkin's disease.
- **Ifosfamide (Ifex):** Non-vesicant, for treatment of lung, hormone-associated cancers, sarcoma, or non-Hodgkin's lymphoma.

61

- **Mechlorethamine hydrochloride (Mustargen):** Vesicant, for treatment of chronic lymphocytic or myelogenous leukemia or Hodgkin's disease.
- **Thiotepa (Thioplex):** Non-vesicant, used before bone marrow transplantation, and to treat Hodgkin's disease, lymphoma, or brain, breast, ovarian or bladder cancers.

VINCA ALKALOIDS

Vinca, or plant-derived, alkaloids inhibit mitosis and are therefore agents that inhibit cell division. There are 3 vinca alkaloids, all vesicants, which are commonly administered. These are vinblastine (Velban), vincristine (Oncovin), and vinorelbine (Navelbine):

- Currently, **vinblastine** is indicated for histiocytosis, Hodgkin's disease, Kaposi's sarcoma, testicular cancer and squamous cell head or neck carcinoma.
- **Vincristine** is used to treat a number of leukemias and lymphomas as well as melanoma, sarcoma, Wilms' tumor, multiple myeloma, neuroblastoma, breast and small cell lung carcinoma.
- **Vinorelbine** is normally used to treat either breast cancer or non-small cell lung cancer.

Each of these agents can cause neurological complications among other side effects. Vinblastine and vinorelbine can also suppress the bone marrow.

ANTITUMOR ANTIBIOTICS

The following are commonly used types of **antitumor antibiotics** by generic and brand name:

- **Bleomycin (Blenoxane):** A non-vesicant, used to treat Hodgkin's disease, non-Hodgkin's lymphoma, head and neck squamous cell carcinomas, and various cancers of the reproductive system.
- **Dactinomycin (Cosmegen):** Vesicant, for treating Wilms' tumor, choriocarcinoma, several connective tissue-derived tumors, or testicular tumors.
- **Daunorubicin hydrochloride (Cerubidine):** Vesicant, used to treat leukemias, especially in children, or non-Hodgkin's lymphoma.
- **Doxorubicin hydrochloride (Adriamycin):** Vesicant, indicated for acute myeloid or lymphocytic leukemias, Hodgkin's disease, small cell lung carcinoma, multiple myeloma, and a variety of other cancers.
- **Doxorubicin Liposome Injection (Doxil):** Irritant, used to treat Kaposi's sarcoma and cancer of the ovaries.
- **Mitomycin (Mutamycin):** Vesicant, for treatment of a wide range of systemic cancers.
- **Mitoxantrone hydrochloride (Novantrone):** Vesicant, indicated primarily for treatment of breast cancer, lymphoma or acute nonlymphocytic leukemia.
- **Plicamycin (Mithracin):** Irritant, used mostly to treat testicular cancer, and the high levels of calcium that may be associated with malignant disease.

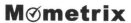

CELL CYCLE-NONSPECIFIC ANTITUMOR AGENTS

Besides alkylating agents and antitumor antibiotics, **nitrosoureas** and **taxanes** are sometimes administered. These agents are not cell cycle specific:

- The **nitrosoureas** include carmustine (BCNU)and streptozocin (Zanosar). BCNU is an irritant and is before bone marrow transplantation, in Hodgkin's and non-Hodgkin's lymphoma, melanoma, myeloma and tumors of the central nervous system.
- **Taxanes** are another classification of agent employed; the most common is docetaxel (Taxotere), which is again an irritant and is indicated for non-small cell lung cancer, ovarian cancer that has metastasized, and cancers of the breast, head and neck regions.

MISCELLANEOUS OR UNIQUE CLASSIFICATIONS OF CELL CYCLE-SPECIFIC ANTITUMOR AGENTS

At present, there are **three common cell cycle-specific agents** that one would put in a **miscellaneous** category. They are asparaginase (Elspar) which is primarily used to treat acute lymphocytic leukemia, irinotecan (Camptosar), commonly used to treat colon or rectal cancer, and paclitaxel (Taxol). Taxol, which can be an irritant, is employed to treat a number of types of cancers, including metastatic ovarian, breast, lung, head, and neck carcinomas as well Kaposi's sarcoma. Another drug called etoposide (VP-16, VePesid) is classified as an epipodophyllotoxin and is commonly used to treat lymphomas and leukemias as well as myeloma, small cell lung cancer, and breast and testicular cancer. Topotecan or Hycamtin is classified as a camptothecin, and it used to treat acute lymphocytic leukemia, metastatic ovarian cancer, some solid tumors as well as non-small cell lung carcinoma.

NOMOGRAM CHART

A **nomogram chart** is a method of calculating body surface area (BSA). There are different charts for adults versus children and infants. BSA in m² (square meters) is determined from the nomogram chart by drawing a line between two scales for height and weight through a scale for body surface area in the middle. The point where the drawn line intersects the body surface scale gives the BSA. Then the antitumor treatment dose is determined by the formula:

Treatment dose (in mg) = Body surface area (in m²) x dose ordered (in mg/m²)

There is also usually lifetime dosage limit for these drugs, which can be calculated by:

Lifetime dose (in mg) = Body surface area (in m²) x recommended limit (in mg/m²)

ANTIMETABOLITES USED FOR CANCER TREATMENT

There are **five main antimetabolites** currently used to treat neoplasms. Each one acts by inhibiting either DNA or protein synthesis by a replacement type of reaction during the actual cell division cycle. Several of these agents are used to treat lymphomas or leukemias, including cytarabine (cytosine arabinoside or Cytosar-U), fludarabine (Fludara), and methotrexate (Mexate-AQ). Methotrexate is indicated for treatment of other cancers as well, including osteogenic sarcoma, gestational trophoblastic tumors, and breast, cervical, lung, head and neck cancers. Two other antimetabolites are also currently used; they are fluorouracil (5-FU) and gemcitabine (Gemzar). Both are employed to treat breast, ovarian, and pancreatic cancer. 5-FU is sometimes used for gastrointestinal tract or liver cancer as well and Gemzar may be given to lung cancer patients. All of these agents are non-vesicants.

CALCULATING ABSOLUTE NEUTROPHIL COUNT

The **absolute neutrophil count (ANC)** is really the primary value that can determine a patient's susceptibility to infection. The ANC is calculated as follows:

ANC (in cells/mm³) = white blood cells (in cells/mm³) x (% polys or segs + % bands)

Normally, the absolute neutrophil count should range from about 3000 to 7000 cells/mm³, but if the ANC is low treatment may be put on hold. Neutropenia is a condition where the ANC is low, equal to or less than 2000 cells/mm³, and in severe cases of neutropenia the count can be less than 500.

TREATMENT GOALS OF ANTINEOPLASTIC THERAPY

When antineoplastic therapy is administered to a patient, the **ultimate goal** is to actually cure the individual, which is defined as a complete response to the therapy where the patient is shown to be completely disease-free for a period of at least 5 years. There can also be less aggressive goals for this therapy. One goal could be to somewhat control the patient's cancer by preventing metastases or prolonging their survival time. Sometimes, the goal is simply to alleviate symptoms without actually curing the underlying disease, known as palliation, which hopefully provides comfort to the patient and may lessen the severity of their symptoms.

SPECIAL INSTRUCTIONS FOR CHEMOTHERAPY PATIENTS DURING TREATMENT COURSE

The health care professional should instruct the chemotherapy patient to self-monitor certain medications, exposures and conditions. The patient should be told to take precautions against possible infection and bleeding. Notably, the patient should avoid aspirin and products that contain aspirin because they could promote bleeding. The patient should make sure they have a sufficient fluid intake including nutritional support products; they should avoid exposure to the sun, be careful about their dental health, and conserve their energy. They should be instructed on how to administer their medications for prevention of vomiting and diarrhea at home. The patient should be advised as to the course of their chemotherapy regimen such as the number of cycles and when they will be administered as well as how this regimen will coordinate with possible concomitant radiation therapy and laboratory testing that may be required.

VEIN SELECTION FOR ANTINEOPLASTIC THERAPY

When **selecting what vein** to administer antineoplastic therapy, one must first consider the areas to avoid. These areas include any place where circulation might have been restricted including veins that are distal to previous venipunctures. Usually it is not recommended to use veins in the joints or hands. If the patient has had a mastectomy or axillary lymph node dissection, sites on that side of the body should be avoided. If they have received radiation therapy on an extremity of their upper body, the side of radiation therapy should be avoided as well. Do not select veins in areas that show bruising or inflammation. If it is possible in light of the other considerations, change the arm to use to insert the catheter.

CHEMOTHERAPY CATHETERS TYPES

Catheters can be inserted short-term, long-term, or even implanted. A **short-term catheter**, where chemotherapy might be needed for only about a month or two, would typically be inserted either into the neck into a jugular vein or under the collar bone with the catheter tip being located in the superior vena cava (SVC). This type of catheter might also be inserted more distally into veins in certain bones but the tip is still located in the SVC.

When extended therapy is needed, one needs to prevent infection and to ensure the catheter stays in place. Such **long-term catheters** often have Dacron cuffs and are inserted under the skin with the tip still in the SVC.

If a patient has limited vascular access, needs lengthy treatment or cannot attend to the catheter, an **implanted catheter** and **port** may be utilized. In this case, there is similar percutaneous insertion but the catheter has an attached reservoir, which is inserted under the skin.

PROTOCOLS FOR ADMINISTERING CHEMOTHERAPY

Protocols for chemotherapy include the following:

- Chemotherapy is typically given orally or with an intravenous catheter.
- Administration could be intermittent where the agent is given at indicated intervals or it could be continuously given for a certain period of time.
- In instances where an intravenous catheter is used, administration can be achieved through a direct IV push with manual pressure or similar pressure through the port of an administration kit.

A couple of **other methods** can be used to **achieve high concentrations** of the medicine at the tumor site.

- The first is use of a catheter put into an artery or an implanted pump with a catheter put into the hepatic artery; this is usually employed in cases of liver disease that has metastasized.
- In addition, sometimes the physician may either surgically implant a reservoir into the area of the cerebrospinal fluid with the catheter placed into the ventricle or he may do a lumbar puncture; these are called intrathecal or intraventricular administrations.

65

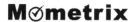

Biologic Therapy

BIOTHERAPY AND IMMUNOTHERAPY

Biotherapy is the use of some type of substance obtained or derived from an actual biologic source. **Immunotherapy** is a form of treatment that utilizes the body's immune processes in some manner. For cancer therapy, commonly employed immunotherapeutic agents fall into three types, interferons, interleukins, and monoclonal antibodies:

- **Interferons** are antiviral substances produced in mammals. Interleukins act by regulating the immune cascade sequence at some point.
- A commonly administered **interleukin** is interleukin-2 (aldesleukin, Proleukin), which is used to treat renal cell carcinoma or metastatic melanoma; one must watch for flu-like symptoms, bone marrow suppression or other side effects.
- **Monoclonal antibodies** have been specifically engineered to react with a particular antigen usually specific to one type of cancer. Currently employed monoclonal antibodies include rituximab (Rituxan), indicated to target CD20+ (a B cell marker) non-Hodgkin's lymphoma, and trastuzumab (Herceptin), which recognizes the HER-2 protein found in some breast carcinomas.

BIOLOGIC AGENTS FOR CANCER TREATMENT

The **three classes of biologic agents** used at present in cancer treatment are hematopoietic growth factors, interferons and interleukins, and monoclonal antibodies.

- **Hematopoietic growth factors** are involved in the development of red blood cells.
- **Interferons** and **interleukins** both have effects on the immune system that can be antiviral or in some way immunomodulatory. Interleukins such as interleukin-2 can actually interfere with tumor cell development and spread.
- **Monoclonal antibodies** are highly specific antibodies that have been developed and isolated to react with specific tumor-associated antigens. These include rituximab and trastuzumab.

INFUSION OF MONOCLONAL ANTIBODIES

Monoclonal antibodies, such as infliximab (Remicade®), bevacizumab (Avastin®), and cetuximab (Erbitux®), are synthesized using DNA technology. Monoclonal antibodies, which are immunosuppressives, are used in the treatment of many types of cancer (usually in combination with other drugs), inflammatory diseases (such as rheumatoid arthritis), multiple sclerosis, and organ transplantation. For cancer treatments, monoclonal antibodies target cancer cells rather than all body cells; however, monoclonal antibodies are associated with a wide range of adverse effects, such as flu-like symptoms (fever, chills, respiratory infections). Primary adverse effects vary according to the specific drug. For example, infliximab may cause headache, rash, GI upset, and upper and lower respiratory infection. Bevacizumab may cause DVT, hypertension, GI upset, leukopenia, hypokalemia, and proteinuria. Patients receiving intravenous infusions of monoclonal antibodies are at increased risk of severe allergic reactions to the drugs. To reduce risk, patients may be premedicated with acetaminophen and diphenhydramine. These same drugs as well as corticosteroids and epinephrine may be used to treat allergic reactions.

INFUSION OF B-CELL INHIBITORS

B-cell inhibitors, such as rituximab (Rituxan®) and tositumomab, are monoclonal antibodies that target and bind to CD20 antigens on B lymphocyte cells (both normal and malignant) and result in destruction of the cell. B-cell inhibitors are used in the treatment of non-Hodgkin's lymphoma

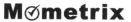

because >90% of B-cell NH lymphomas express the CD20 antigens, so destruction of these cells decreases the malignant cells. In other diseases, such as rheumatoid arthritis, the destruction of B-cells decreases the production of autoantibodies, reducing the effects of the disease. Rituximab may cause tumor lysis syndrome with acute renal failure, respiratory distress syndrome, flu-like symptoms, dyspnea, bronchospasm, and pulmonary infiltrates. Tositumomab may cause flu-like symptoms, headache, rash, infection, and hypertension. As with other monoclonal antibodies, patients who are to receive B-cell inhibitors per IV infusion should be premedicated with acetaminophen and diphenhydramine to prevent severe and sometimes fatal allergic reactions.

INFUSION OF T-CELL INHIBITORS

T-cell inhibitors, such as abatacept (Orencia®), are immunomodulating drugs that inhibit T-cell activation. Abatacept is used primarily in the treatment of rheumatoid arthritis and may be used in conjunction with other DMARDs or by itself if DMARDs have been infective. Intravenous infusions are given initially and at 2-week intervals for the first month of treatment and then once a month, with dosage according to patient's weight in Kg. The infusion is usually per intravenous infusion administered over a 30-minute period with an IV filter in place. Adverse effects include cold and flu-like symptoms, and hypertension. Patients should not receive vaccinations while being treated with T-cell inhibitors, especially live vaccines, and should not receive anakinra, TNF-blocking drugs, or echinacea because of increased risk of infection. Because of the risk (rare) of severe allergic reactions, patients should be premedicated with acetaminophen and diphenhydramine.

IMMUNE MODULATOR REAGENTS

Immune modulator agents can be compounds that stimulate or suppress the immune system, or they may be targeted monoclonal antibodies. The most common immunostimulant is probably immune globulin IV (Sandoglobulin is a commercial name), which is used to restore immunoglobulin G levels. There are several agents available that suppress the immune system. These include aldesleukin (Interleukin-2 Recombinant), often given to patients with cancer or some other type of immune malfunction, azathioprine sodium (Imuran), and cyclosporine (Sandimmune IV), which is administered before transplantation surgery. Monoclonal antibodies are antibodies that are isolated or produced with a targeted specificity. Today they are used to treat a number of diseases, including alemtuzumab (Campath), which is employed to treat leukemia.

67

Anti-Infective Infusions

PENICILLINS

Penicillin is an antibiotic that was originally isolated from mold but now has many synthetic forms including the following:

- **Ampicillin sodium (Omnipen-N):** Used to treat both gram-positive and negative bacteria, excluding staphylococci that produce penicillinase.
- **Nafcillin sodium (Unipen):** To treat staphylococci that generate penicillinase.
- **Oxacillin sodium (Bactocill):** Indicated for penicillinase-producing bacteria.
- **Penicillin G potassium/sodium:** For serious infections including anaerobic ones and those affecting the heart or brain.
- **Piperacillin sodium (Pipracil):** Used to treat organisms affecting the respiratory or urinary tracts as well as solid areas such as the bones.
- **Ticarcillin disodium (Ticar):** Broad spectrum penicillin to treat bacterial infections that have become septicemic.

CEPHALOSPORINS

Currently available **cephalosporins** are generally given to treat gram-negative, gram-positive or occasionally anaerobic infections that do not require oxygen. Any generic drug name with a *cef-* prefix is probably a cephalosporin. Broad-spectrum cephalosporins include cefazolin sodium (Kefzol), cefamandole nafate (Mandol), cefotetan disodium (Cefotan), cefuroxime sodium (Kefurox) and others. Some cephalosporins are usually employed to treat bacterial infections in specific body areas, typically on the skin or bones, genitalia, urinary tract, or respiratory tract. Examples include cephapirin sodium (Cefadyl) and ceftizoxime sodium (Cefizox).

RELATIONSHIP BETWEEN PENICILLINS AND CEPHALOSPORINS

Cephalosporin was originally isolated from a mold just like penicillin and is very similar in structure. Cephalosporins, which now include a variety of further generation derivatives, are more resistant than penicillins to the action of penicillinase. Because of their similar structure, some of the cephalosporins can cross-react in a patient with penicillin allergy and therefore be contraindicated. Cephalosporins are generally effective against gram-positive, gram-negative and often anaerobic bacteria.

AMINOGLYCOSIDES

Aminoglycosides are antibiotics that structurally have their amino sugars attached as glycosides. Their primary use is to treat infections caused by aerobic bacilli. Bacilli are rod-shaped, spore-forming bacteria. They include *Escherichia coli, Klebsiella*, and *Pseudomonas*, and *Proteus* species. Some aminoglycosides are effective against both gram stain-negative and gram-positive bacilli, and these include gentamicin sulfate (Garamycin), netilmicin sulfate (Netromycin), and Tobramycin sulfate (Nebcin). Some are effective against primarily gram-negative organisms, including kanamycin sulfate (Kantrex) and amikacin sulfate (Amikin).

TETRACYCLINE

A **tetracycline** is a type of antibiotic whose structure contains four rings. It is effective because it inhibits protein synthesis by inhibiting the binding of transfer RNA. Tetracyclines are broad-spectrum reagents that can inhibit the growth of both gram-positive as well as gram-negative bacteria as well as rickettsiae, *Chlamydia*, and *Mycoplasma pneumoniae*. The most commonly used

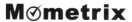

tetracycline is doxycycline hyclate (Vibramycin IV). Side effects of Vibramycin can include skin rashes and photosensitivity so the patient should be instructed to avoid sun exposure.

ERYTHROMYCINS

Erythromycins are a type of antibiotic effective against gram-positive organisms. Originally, erythromycin was isolated from *Streptomyces erythreus.* Today, erythromycin lactobionate (Erythrocin) is commonly given and indicated for treatment of staphylococci, pneumococci, or streptococci. It is usually administered at a dosage of 15 to 20 mg/kg per day. Major side effects can be hives, phlebitis, or pain along the vein.

ANTIFUNGAL AGENTS

Common **antifungal drugs** include the following:

- **Amphotericin B (Fungizone)**: given to treat fungal infections that have invaded the patient's whole body
- **Fluconazole (Diflucan)**: for treatment of *Candida*, infections with cryptococcus, or some systemic infections
- **Miconazole (Monistat IV)**: specifically used to combat *Candida, Cryptococcus neoformans*, or *Aspergillus fumigatus*

A special note would be that Amphotericin B, given usually at a dose of 10 mg/250 mL over 4 hours by slow infusion, needs to first prepared in preservative-free sterile water followed by dilution in 5% dextrose in water and then filtered and protected from the light.

AGENTS WITH ANTIVIRAL PROPERTIES

Antibiotics are not effective in treating viral infections. There are, however, a few agents with **antiviral properties**; their principal mode of action is to block or inhibit replication of viral DNA. All of these drugs are given intermittently. Current antiviral drugs include acyclovir sodium (Zovirax), which is used to treat herpes simplex infections; foscarnet sodium (Foscavir), which is useful to reduce the viral load in acyclovir-resistant herpes or cytomegalovirus infections; ganciclovir sodium (Cytovene, DHPG), indicated for eye infections with cytomegalovirus, herpes or Epstein-Barr virus; and zidovudine (AZT, Retrovir), which is the primarily drug used to treat patients with human immunodeficiency virus (HIV).

PROTOZOA

Protozoa are unicellular, non-photosynthetic, flagellated organisms. They are parasites, meaning they have some sort of symbiotic relationship with their host, in this case the human body. Currently available antiprotozoals include metronidazole hydrochloride (Flagyl I.V.), usually utilized for severe skin, bone, or joint infections, and pentamidine isethionate (Pentam 300), and usually indicated for Pneumocystis carinii type of pneumonia. The latter is also used as an investigational drug for some other protozoal diseases such as sleeping sickness.

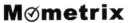

MISCELLANEOUS TYPES OF ANTIBIOTICS

The following are some **miscellaneous types of antibiotics** that might be chosen for unique conditions:

- **Chloramphenicol sodium succinate** (Chloromycetin) is indicated for mild cases of bacterial infection in the blood and also for patients with Rocky Mountain spotted fever or cystic fibrosis.
- **Vancomycin hydrochloride** (Vancocin HCL Intravenous) is given to treat gram-positive cocci.
- **Quinolones**, such as levofloxacin (Levaquin) are indicated for respiratory tract infections.
- **Co-trimoxazole** (Bactrim IV Infusion) is a combination of antibiotics of the sulfonamide type, and is used to treat serious urinary tract infections.

ANTIGENS AND ANTIBODIES

Normally an **antigen** is a substance that is recognized as foreign by the body that is then likely to induce an immune response or production of antibodies. **Antibodies** are protein molecules that react specifically with the inducing antigen. In the case of red blood cells, there are inherited glycoprotein or glycolipid antigens found on the cell surface. These antigens can produce an immune response in which antibodies are produced. In the presence of red cells with the corresponding antigen, a process called agglutination can occur in which the cells clump. Therefore, one must know the antigens present on the red cell before transfusion to avoid this reaction. The study of these immune responses in the blood is known as immunohematology.

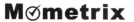

Blood Transfusions

ABO Blood Group System

On the red cell, there can be antigens called **A and B, a combination of both (AB), or none (O).** Most individuals have been typed for these antigens, and blood components to be transfused have as well. If the antigen is present on the red cell, then it is not foreign and no antibodies are present; if the antigen is not present, antibodies will be found. Therefore, **the most universal type of blood to transfuse is group O** which has both anti-A and anti-B antibodies; group O patients must receive this type. Group A patients have antibodies to group B, so they can only receive red cells from either groups A or O. Group B patients have plasma antibodies to group A and can only be transfused with groups B or O. Since those typed as **group AB** have both antigens on the red cell but no corresponding circulating antibodies, they can receive red cells from any blood group and are called **universal recipients**.

Rh Factor

In addition to the ABO blood group, blood is generally typed for Rh factor. **Rh factor** is another antigen found on red blood cells. While there are about 50 identified Rh antigens, an antigen called D is the most important. If a patient has antigen D on their red cells, they are classified as Rh-positive, and conversely if antigen D is absent, the individual is Rh-negative. Rh-negative blood can be given to anyone, but if Rh-positive blood is administered to Rh-negative individuals, antibodies will be produced which is undesirable. The Rh status of the patient and donor blood is crucial for transfusing patients of childbearing age to obviate the possibility of complications if they become pregnant.

Isolating Various Blood Components

If blood loss can be replaced with blood components and crystalloid or colloid solutions, usually **whole blood transfusion** is not indicated. However, during an episode of acute and significant blood loss, the patient may have pulmonary and heart problems plus a low hematocrit. This means oxygen-carrying capacity is diminished because of low red cell count and the blood volume is low, which can lead to shock. The whole blood is transfused as rapidly as possible mainly to increase the volume and resolve symptoms of hypovolemic shock. The blood must be ABO compatible.

Infusion of Isolated Red Blood Cells

Red blood cells (RBCs) that have been separated from the plasma are generally administered to the patient in cases where it is necessary to increase or maintain the oxygen-carrying ability of the blood, but an actual increase in blood volume is not needed. RBCs can be used to treat symptoms of anemia that have not responded to other treatments. Sometimes hypovolemic shock can be managed with RBCs and crystalloid or protein solutions. RBCs should be infused within 4 hours of onset of symptoms. They may require dilution with 0.9% saline because they may be very viscous if anticoagulants or preservatives have been added. ABO compatibility must be considered.

Leukocyte-Reduced RBCs

Red blood cells can be washed within 24 hours of the transfusion time, which reduces the number of RBCs by about 20%. More often, RBCs are actually filtered during processing or at the patient's bedside, and as much as 99% of the leukocytes can be removed from the preparation by this type of procedure. A unit of **leukocyte-reduced RBCs** has fewer than 500 million leukocytes. Use of these leukocyte-reduced RBCs is indicated in cases where the patient is known to react to white cell donor antigens or in immunosuppressed patients. They may also be used to diminish the possibility or skin or anaphylactic reactions, to prevent transmission of cytomegalovirus, or to prevent development of antibodies to leukocyte antigens.

71

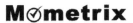

FRESH FROZEN PLASMA PREPARATIONS

Fresh frozen plasma, which is prepared by separating the plasma from the cells, contains a variety of proteins including albumin, antibodies, and other proteins. It also contains clotting factors, which is the main reason plasma is chosen for transfusion. Plasma transfusion is chosen for patients who have demonstrated a deficiency in the level of clotting factors to increase that level; it is not indicated as a method to increase the volume or as a protein nutritional supplement. Coagulation response should be improved with this therapy. Plasma administration can also neutralize the anticoagulant effects of warfarin therapy. Clotting factors V and VIII can be destroyed if the plasma is not infused within 24 hours of thawing.

PLATELETS

Platelets are sometimes transfused into a patient. Platelets, or thrombocytes, are plasma components obtained by separation that are important in the clotting process. Platelet transfusion is useful in cases of thrombocytopenia or atypical platelet function to prevent or stop bleeding and increase the platelet count. Platelets are prepared by collecting the blood and separating the platelets from the plasma and then usually pooling of donors into a single bag; sometimes an individual donor is used. They should be stored with gentle rotation for up to 5 days before use. The main advantage of using platelets is that the ABO blood type is irrelevant; however, ABO typing is still recommended to reduce the potential for resistance to the platelets.

HLA

HLA means **human leukocyte antigen**, which is an antigen found on the white cell surface. Antibodies can form against this antigen in patients and these HLA antibodies can cause early destruction of transferred platelets. If HLA-matched platelets are used, this decreases the possibility of their destruction after transfusion. HLA-matched platelets are most commonly obtained from a family member but sometimes other donors will have fairly good matches and can be used. HLA-matched platelets are most commonly used for patients who will be undergoing tissue or organ transplantation. Reduction of leukocytes by filtration can also help prevent HLA alloimmunization.

INDIVIDUAL BLEEDING FACTORS

The most common types of **individual bleeding factors** that might be used in transfusion therapy are factor VIII and factor IX, useful for patients with hemophilia A and B respectively. Factor VIII concentrates are usually used when there is either ongoing bleeding or prophylactically in a patient who has been determined to be factor VIII deficient (hemophilia A). Some of the newer preparations also have activity against von Willebrand's disease. These concentrates need to reconstituted and then administered within 3 hours. Patients classified as hemophilia B, also known as Christmas disease, are deficient in factor IX. Again, the factor IX concentrate is reconstituted and diluted. In this case, the half-life of the infused factor IX is very short, so formulas given for the amount to administer should usually be increased twofold. The goal of either factor is to stop the bleeding, and because they are both purified concentrates antigen compatibility does not need to considered.

CRYOPRECIPITATE

A **cryoprecipitate** is a component usually isolated from a single unit of fresh frozen plasma. It contains several factors involved in the bleeding cascade including factor VIII (anti-hemophilia factor), von Willebrand's factor, and factor XIII. Cryoprecipitate is sometimes used if any of these factors or fibrinogen are deficient to reduce or stop bleeding. ABO and Rh factor matching of the donor is usually preferred as well. The unit or pooled units of cryoprecipitate have to be infused

72

within 6 or 4 hours respectively after thawing. Therefore, while after laboratory evaluation a dose can be repeated in 8 to 12 hours, a newly thawed unit must be used. Units often need to be diluted with 0.9% saline in order to infuse them.

COLLOID SOLUTIONS

The two common types of **colloid solutions** that might be transfused are both basically protein solutions that have been commercially extracted from plasma solutions. They are either albumin or the protein plasma fraction. They are used most often to treat low protein levels. In some cases, the albumin solution is actually used as a plasma substitute when there is massive hemorrhage or shock due to low plasma volume. Both types of solutions should increase the plasma volume expansion and prevent considerable concentration of the blood. They may also decrease the possibility of edema in the patient and increase their serum protein levels.

AUTOLOGOUS TRANSFUSION

Autologous transfusion is the process of transfusing the patient's own blood or components that have been collected and labeled at least 3 days prior to surgery. This ensures that the transfused blood contains red cells of the same allotype, which basically means the antigens recognized will be specific for that patient. Intraoperative auto transfusion is another type of autologous transfusion where the blood must be collected and then reinfused within 8 hours of collection using good aseptic technique. If there is a possibility of excessive bacterial contamination or presence of malignant cells, this procedure is usually contraindicated. Usually this is only done if at least 3 units of blood can be retransfused. Occasionally, there is a similar procedure called postoperative blood salvage that is done, where blood is collected right after surgery for possible reinfusion up to 6 hours later.

PRE-TRANSFUSION PATIENT HISTORY

Evaluations of the patient should be done before considering transfusion therapy. A **patient history** including current and continual conditions or medications, prior transfusion history, and religious or cultural beliefs should be taken before considering transfusion. Clinical vital signs should be evaluated including renal and venous status. Laboratory tests should be done prior to infusion including a hematocrit, hemoglobin levels, evaluation of platelets, electrolyte levels, liver function tests, and assays for albumin, clotting factors, and serum iron binding capacity. Additionally, the patient's mental capacity at the time should be assessed.

VASCULAR ACCESS DEVICES AND BLOOD ADMINISTRATION SETS EMPLOYED DURING TRANSFUSION

In most patients, an 18- or 20-gauge catheter is connected to a large vein as a vascular access device but sometimes a smaller gauge catheter is used in children or adults without accessible large veins. **Blood administration sets** come in four types:

- A **straight blood administration set** may be used if only an individual unit is to be given.
- If multiple units are to be transfused, a **Y-type set** would generally be used, in which one arm of the Y contains 0.9% saline while the other side delivers the blood.
- If platelets or cryoprecipitate are to be administered, a **component recipient set** may be used to reduce the possibility of cell destruction; the set is shorter and has a smaller filter.
- There is also a type of set called a **component infusion set,** which makes it easier to directly push the component intravenously.

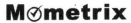

FILTERS CONNECTED TO BLOOD ADMINISTRATION SETS

Filters are often an integral part of blood administration sets or they may be added. Their main function is to prevent passage of clots or other materials found in the blood or blood components being transfused. The size of a standard filter is usually from 170 to 260 microns; nothing larger than that size will pass through the filter. However, microaggregate filters with smaller pore sizes of 20 to 40 microns are recommended when administering whole blood or packed cells that have been stored for 5 or more days or for patients undergoing bypass surgery. There are also filters that will remove essentially all of the leukocytes in a component.

EXTERNAL DEVICES USED DURING TRANSFUSION

External devices that might be utilized during transfusion include:

- **An electronic infusion device**: Basically an external pump, regulated by pressure (psi); must be monitored to prevent cell damage.
- **An external pressure cuff**: A cuff with a gauge to monitor pressure (not to exceed 300 mmHg), used primarily during rapid administration.
- **A blood or fluid warmer**: A warm water bath or electric heated plate device that can increase the temperature of the blood or RBCs being infused; generally used during large infusions of blood that has been refrigerated or in newborns or patients with known cold agglutinins.

ACUTE HEMOLYTIC REACTIONS

Acute hemolytic reactions to transfusion therapy can be either intravascular or extravascular. They are both caused by incompatibilities between donor and recipient blood components. Intravascular reactions are generally caused by donor red blood cells that are ABO incompatible with the recipient's plasma and extravascular events are usually a result of donor plasma that is mismatched for the recipient's red blood cells. In either case, fever and chills can occur although it may be several hours later for extravascular events. For acute intravascular hemolytic reactions, the patient may have other evidence of abnormal bleeding, pain or possibly leading to shock. In either case, stop transfusion immediately, administer 0.9% sodium chloride instead, notify the physician and blood bank, and start treatments to reverse the adverse effects.

DELAYED ONSET ALLOIMMUNIZATION

Days or even years after transfusion, delayed adverse reactions can occur. There are antigens on red blood cells in addition to the ABO system antigens. These include not only the Rh antigens but the Kell, Duffy and Kidd antigens among others. A patient can have a **delayed sensitivity reaction** to these antigens if they are foreign and present on the donor's red blood cells. This is known as primary alloimmunization. If a patient is exposed again to foreign antigens, resulting in further antibody production, they may develop a state of secondary alloimmunization. In either case, symptoms could include an unexplained fever, a drop in hemoglobin levels, mild jaundice or presence of hemoglobin in the urine. Renal function must be monitored. The foreign antigen should be identified to avoid its use in future transfusions.

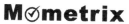

TRANSFUSION-TRANSMITTED VIRUSES

Viral infections can be transmitted during transfusion and produce delayed onset adverse reactions. The most common types of **transfusion-transmitted viruses** include:

- **Hepatitis B or Hepatitis C**: Associated with post-transfusion liver function abnormalities occurring up to about 6 months after transfusion, and presenting with fatigue, nausea or jaundice.
- **Human T-cell lymphotropic virus (HTLV)**: Associated with acquired immunodeficiency, in particular HTLV-III also known as HIV which causes AIDS; this facilitates the growth of opportunistic infections, and symptoms may include fever, night sweats, skin lesions or enlarged lymph nodes.
- **Cytomegalovirus**: Member of herpes virus family sometimes causing symptoms similar to mononucleosis but usually asymptomatic; however, associated morbidity and death can occur in immunocompromised patients.

GRAFT VERSUS HOST DISEASE

Graft versus host disease is a condition that can occur in an immunosuppressed patient when they are transfused with immunocompetent lymphocytes. It is basically a delayed onset reaction to the antigens on the donor's immunocompetent lymphocytes where host tissues are destroyed because the patient cannot mount a normal immunological response. The term is often associated with transplantation and rejection of grafts. In the case of transfusions, the patient usually becomes feverish and may develop rashes, hepatitis, or diarrhea. Because the patient does not have normal immune function, the disease can lead to suppression of the bone marrow, which facilitates massive infection, which can result in death. If the blood components are irradiated prior to transfusion, this disease can often be eliminated in immunosuppressed patients.

FEBRILE NONHEMOLYTIC REACTIONS

Sometimes a patient being transfused presents with a slight increase in temperature (1-2 °F) during transfusion or after its completion. This temperature increase may be accompanied by chills or general fatigue. This is known as a **febrile nonhemolytic reaction** and is caused by an antigen-antibody reaction in the white blood cells. Transfusion should be stopped and changed to 0.9% saline, the physician and blood bank should be notified, and drugs to reduce fever should be administered. Blood donor products that have been leukocyte-reduced will help prevent this type of reaction. If the patient has a history of these types of reactions, they can be medicated beforehand.

ALLERGIC REACTION

An **allergic reaction** is a harmful type of reaction to a foreign protein, resulting in sensitivity to that protein. During transfusion, the foreign protein or antigen is generally some type of plasma protein from the donor. The reaction could be mild, more severe, or even life-threatening, such as anaphylactic shock. Allergic reactions that are less severe usually manifest themselves as some sort of skin reaction, such as hives or local redness. The transfusion should be interrupted and antihistamines administered for mild reactions; sometimes the transfusion can be later restarted. If the reaction is more severe, the doctor should be called. Anaphylaxis is a very severe allergic reaction involving the respiratory system. The patient goes into respiratory distress, has bronchospasm, and may have gastrointestinal issues as well. Anaphylaxis can proceed to shock, unconsciousness, and death so it must be attended to immediately. Stop transfusion, notify the doctor and blood bank, and initiate anti-allergic treatment.

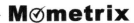

ADVERSE REACTIONS THAT MIGHT OCCUR IF INFUSED TOO RAPIDLY

If a patient with less than ideal cardiac or pulmonary status is **infused too rapidly**, circulatory overload may occur. The patient may present with pulmonary edema problems such as difficulty breathing, or circulation issues such as headache, cyanosis, hypertension or even congestive heart failure. Generally, the transfusion should be stopped and the patient should be put into a sitting position and diuretics and/or oxygen given. If refrigerated blood or its components are administered to any type of patient, hypothermia can occur; symptoms of the patient could include chills, hypotension or cardiac arrhythmia. If measures to warm the blood are begun and treatment of symptoms initiated, the transfusion may usually proceed.

INFUSION OF CONTAMINATED BLOOD COMPONENT

Although rare, sometimes bacteria can be introduced during infusion. This is generally due to the presence of gram-negative organisms in the components. Use of good aseptic technique from collection, through processing, and during administration of the blood products should prevent this. However, if it does occur, the patient may present with a high fever, skin that is red or hot, hypotension, shock, renal failure, or widespread intravascular coagulation. Measures to prevent shock should be initiated as soon as possible, the doctor and blood bank should be notified, the transfusion should be terminated, and the administration set should be switched to 0.9% sodium chloride. All suspected avenues of contamination should be cultured including the patient's own blood, the transfused product, mechanical components, and the saline solution.

UNIQUE ADVERSE REACTIONS TO TRANSFUSIONS IN PATIENTS WITH LIVER IMPAIRMENT

Patients with **liver impairment** cannot metabolize citrate in their liver. When these patients are given a large volume transfusion, a condition called citrate toxicity can occur because of their inability to metabolize citrate. The recipient may present with tingling of the lips, hypotension, nausea, vomiting, and cardiac arrhythmia. They may also have low levels of calcium or potassium. Therefore, if the transfusion is continued at a slower rate, serum calcium and potassium levels must be monitored. It is essential to know the patient's history of liver impairment before transfusion.

IRON OVERLOAD

A patient who has received many transfusions may develop a condition known as **iron overload** in which iron has been progressively built up in the circulation. The condition occurs most often in recipients with hemoglobin abnormalities. This iron accumulation can lead to liver failure or cardiac toxicity. If iron overload is anticipated or suspected, there are methods to remove the iron without lowering the amount of circulating hemoglobin, and a drug called deferoxamine mesylate can be given.

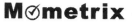

Other Infused Agents

CHELATING AGENTS

Chelating agents are molecules that remove unwanted heavy metal ions from the body by combining with them to form a compound called a chelate. The most common use of a chelating agent would be to remove excess iron. Acute iron intoxication or chronic iron overload is typically treated with the chelating agent called deferoxamine mesylate or Desferal. It is usually administered intramuscularly but may be introduced beneath the skin. The usual dose would be 15 mg/kg/hr. The nurse should frequently take samples to measure serum ferritin or iron concentration as well as blood gases, central venous pressure, and the patient's renal function.

TREATMENT FOR PATHOLOGIC CONDITIONS INVOLVING OVERSECRETION IN GI TRACT

There are 3 common agents utilized in treatment of pathologic conditions characterized by **oversecretion in the gastrointestinal tract.** They are ranitidine (Zantac), cimetidine hydrochloride (Tagamet), and famotidine (Pepcid I.V.). Cimetidine and famotidine are also given to treat ulcers. Cimetidine can enhance the effects of warfarin anticoagulants so prothrombin time and dosage need to be monitored. Abdominal side effects such as diarrhea, nausea and vomiting are more common with Zantac or Pepcid I.V.

AGENTS TO TREAT NAUSEA AND VOMITING

Metoclopramide hydrochloride (Reglan), ondansetron hydrochloride (Zofran), or droperidol (Inapsine) may be administered to treat gastrointestinal problems such as **nausea and vomiting**. Reglan is commonly used as a preventive measure, often before (or after) administering chemotherapy. Inapsine is also used as a sedating agent before surgery so the health care professional should always be watching how conscious the patient remains. The side effects of Zofran are mainly changes in bowel habits.

HORMONES OR SYNTHETIC SUBSTITUTES

The **hormone** insulin is administered continuously intravenously or by push in cases of diabetic coma or ketoacidosis or for short-term management of potassium excess. Serum glucose levels and symptoms of either hypo- or hyperglycemia must be monitored. Glucagon hydrochloride is used to treat hypoglycemia. The hormone oxytocin, known commercially as Pitocin, has a completely different indication. It is used to induce labor or to encourage postpartum contractions in order to decrease bleeding. Side effects to the mother and fetus must be watched, such as rupture of the uterus, fluid retention or hypertension in the mother, or damage to the brain or central nervous system or irregular heartbeats in the child.

SODIUM BICARBONATE

Sodium bicarbonate is sometimes administered either by push or continuously. Indications for its use include asthma attacks, barbiturate intoxication, or metabolic acidosis. Dosage is dependent upon pH, $PaCO_2$, base requirements and fluid restrictions, and may be adjusted during administration. The infusion site should be watched because leaking and subsequent tissue damage can occur. Other side effects could include muscle spasms, hyperexcitability, high pH, headache, nausea, and low potassium levels.

AMINOPHYLLINE

Aminophylline, or theophylline ethylenediamine, is a respiratory smooth muscle relaxant, which is administered either by push or continuously. It is used to treat bronchial asthma or the treatable bronchospasm that is associated with chronic bronchitis or emphysema. Serum drug levels and

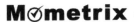

respiratory rate are usually measured periodically if aminophylline is given; it should not be administered too rapidly. Gastrointestinal, neurological, and cardiac side effects can occur.

STEROID INFUSIONS

Steroid infusions with intravenous preparations, such as methylprednisolone and dexamethasone, may be injected slowly directly into a vein or added to 5DW, NS, or 5% D/NS for IV infusion. Steroid infusions may be used for many different conditions, but are commonly used to treat exacerbations or relapses of multiple sclerosis, typically administered daily for 3 days. Steroid infusions may also be used for adrenocortical insufficiency rheumatic disorders (rheumatoid arthritis), collagen diseases (lupus erythematosus), dermatologic diseases (psoriasis), allergic conditions (acute asthma), ophthalmic disease (optic neuritis), hemolytic disorders (ITP), respiratory disease (berylliosis), spinal cord injury, and cancer (palliative treatment of leukemias). Dosage varies depending on the reason for use, but doses must be tapered to avoid steroid withdrawal syndrome. Adverse effects include anxiety, facial hair growth (female), abnormal fat distribution (upper back), weight gain, round face, fluid retention, infections, osteoporosis, aseptic necrosis, flushing, metallic taste in the mouth, GI bleeding, mood changes, insomnia, and hot flashes.

TREATMENT FOR CALCIUM DEFICIENCY

Calcium is administered in its chloride or gluconate forms to treat calcium deficiency or hypocalcemia. Calcium chloride is usually indicated for treatment of muscle spasms that are associated with low calcium levels. Calcium gluconate is generally given when calcium deficiency is caused by vitamin D shortage, but it is also given to counteract the toxic effects of magnesium sulfate or for general electrolyte imbalance. Both of these solutions could produce cardiac side effects or tissue damage as a result of leaking at the injection site. Serum calcium levels should be monitored.

VITAMIN DEFICIENCY SYNDROMES TREATED BY PUSH OR CONTINUOUS ADMINISTRATION OF ANTIDOTES

Multivitamins are sometimes administered continuously if a patient is vitamin deficient. Single vitamins, derivatives, or antidotes for a specific deficiency are also given at times by injection or continuously. Examples include folic acid (Folvite), indicated for megaloblastic anemias resulting from poor nutrition; pyridoxine hydrochloride (Hexa Betalin), to treat vitamin B_6 deficiency; thiamine hydrochloride (Betalin S), if an individual is thiamine deficient; and vitamin K or phytonadione (AquaMEPHYTON), which is used to treat a number of hemolytic or liver-related diseases.

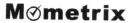

Body Fluid Composition

IMPORTANCE OF BODY FLUIDS IN BODY COMPOSITION AT VARIOUS AGES

Body fluids comprise approximately 80% of body weight in infants. By puberty, adult body weight is generally achieved, at which point fluids account for about 60% of the body weight. Body fluid is excreted in a number of forms including through the pores as sweat, by the kidneys as urine, as water vapor from the lungs, and as vomit and diarrhea from our intestinal tract. Females usually have a lower percentage of fluid weight due to increased storage of fat. Most people also tend to have an increased body fat content with aging and therefore a decrease in relative fluid content.

FLUID COMPARTMENTS IN THE BODY

Body fluids are found as either **intracellular fluid (ICF)** or **extracellular fluid (ECF)**. ICF is the fluid found inside the cells and, in an adult, it comprises the largest proportion of body weight, approximately two thirds. Any fluids outside of the cells are said to be extracellular. Sweat, gastrointestinal secretions, lymph, cerebrospinal fluid, and ocular, pleural, synovial and pericardial fluids are all examples of ECF. Extracellular fluid is further subdivided into two categories: interstitial fluid, which is fluid located between the cells, and intravascular fluid, which is fluid located within the vessels of the vascular system.

ELECTROLYTE

An **electrolyte** is a substance that separates chemically in solution, giving it the ability to then conduct an electrical charge. Electrolytes are either negatively charged particles called anions or positively charged particles called cations. Both anions and cations are found in intracellular fluids (ICF) and extracellular fluids (ECF). In ICF, the principal cation is potassium plus some magnesium and a little sodium, while the primary anion found is phosphate with some sulfate, bicarbonate, and proteinate. In ECF, the most prevalent cation is sodium, while calcium, magnesium, and potassium are also found. The primary anion found in extracellular fluid is chloride, with phosphate, bicarbonate, sulfate, proteinate, and organic acids present in addition. There are also nonelectrolyte solutions in the body such as sugars, fats, and vitamins.

GLANDS AND CORRESPONDING HORMONES THAT EXERT CONTROL OVER FLUID AND ELECTROLYTE BALANCE

One endocrine gland, the **pituitary gland** secretes *antidiuretic hormone (ADH)* when it is stimulated by the hypothalamus in the brain. ADH regulates water excretion and conservation in the kidneys. There are two hormones controlling homeostasis that are secreted from the **adrenal gland**, *aldosterone* and *cortisol*. Both of these hormones facilitate potassium excretion and consequent restoration of fluid volume by building up sodium. The **parathyroid gland** produces *parathyroid hormone*. If levels of this hormone are high then so are calcium levels but conversely phosphate levels are lowered. The **thyroid gland** releases a compound called *calcitonin,* which acts in exactly the opposite way; if calcitonin is present in high concentrations, then calcium is actually decreased.

HOMEOSTASIS AND ORGANS INVOLVED IN FLUID AND ELECTROLYTE BALANCE

Homeostasis is the tendency to reach a state of equilibrium or balance. In the case of fluid and electrolyte balance, the primary regulator of fluid balance is the renal system, specifically the urine output from the kidneys. The cardiac system is directly involved here as well because heart and blood vessels circulate the blood through the kidneys, where urine is produced. In addition, a number of other systems facilitate homeostatic mechanisms to maintain water and electrolyte

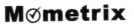

balance. These include the respiratory system in which lungs release water when we exhale and the endocrine system, which contains various glands that control chemical reactions.

EFFECTS OF FLUID VOLUME LEVELS AND ELECTROLYTES ON CARDIAC SYSTEM

The heart and **cardiac system** ultimately push plasma through the kidneys for fluid elimination. Therefore, the pulse is related to fluid volume levels. If fluid volume is low, there is a weak, rapid pulse. Fluid overload will conversely lead to a slow but full pulse. Sodium affects changes in blood volume levels. Potassium stimulates nerve impulses as well as wave generation in the heart muscle. The heart's ability to contract and relax is regulated by calcium. Another electrolyte, magnesium, produces dilation of the blood vessels, which can lead to unwanted effects such as a decrease in blood pressure and possible cardiac shutdown.

AGE GROUPS MOST VULNERABLE TO FLUID OR ELECTROLYTE IMBALANCES

The **most vulnerable age groups** that might experience fluid or electrolyte imbalances are infants and the elderly. Infants do not have a fully developed kidney function, and they generally excrete more than they take in. Therefore, they may experience too low fluid levels. The elderly are at increased risk for a fluid depletion. They often have an inadequate renal function and the respiratory system often cannot maintain a normal pH. It is hard for the health care provider to determine their fluid status because their skin lacks elasticity. The elderly are often confused, they do not feel thirsty enough to drink, or they often are taking diuretics or laxatives, all of which can lead to a net fluid deficit.

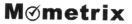

Fluid Volume Excess or Deficit

MEDICATIONS THAT CAN CAUSE FLUID OR ELECTROLYTE IMBALANCES

Several types of **medications or intravenous solutions (IV) can create fluid or electrolyte imbalances:**

- If a patient is taking **diuretics**, fluids and electrolytes are often depleted. Depending on the diuretic used, sometimes there can actually be high electrolyte levels.
- If the individual is taking **laxatives**, they may have low potassium levels.
- Administration of **corticosteroids** often causes fluid and electrolyte accumulation, reduced potassium levels, or abnormally high pH in the respiratory and metabolic systems.
- Certain **IV solutions** can lead to fluid or electrolyte imbalances as well. The most common examples would be excessive administration of sodium-containing solutions, which could result in fluid volume excess or increased sodium levels, or use of electrolyte-free solutions, which could deplete electrolytes.

ASSESSMENT FOR FLUID BALANCE

To clinically **assess the patient for signs of fluid imbalance**, the nurse should first check for fluid ingestion versus excretion and other output. The nurse should confirm urine volume and its concentration. They should check the turgor of the skin and tongue. The health care professional should verify whether the patient is thirsty, tearing, or salivating. Body weight and its fluctuation can also be an indicator of fluid status. Other important measurements include checking for swelling, observing the appearance and temperature of the skin, checking vital signs and central venous pressure, verifying that the oral cavity is moist, and observing whether there are any neurological changes.

VITAL SIGNS

4 vital signs should be regularly documented include temperature, pulse, respiratory rate, and blood pressure:

- A high **temperature** can indicate a fluid volume deficit often caused by excessive sweating, but sometimes a low temperature can indicate a low volume as well.
- **Pulse** measures the heart rate. If there is a low fluid volume the heart rate needs to increase in order to maintain cardiac output. Electrolyte imbalances can affect the heart rate; the rate is increased with low potassium or magnesium or elevated sodium and vice versa. Potassium or magnesium deficiencies can also precipitate an irregular heartbeat.
- A fluid volume deficit or loss can cause an upsurge in the **respiratory rate.** Too much fluid, on the other hand, can be indicated by a shortness of breath or moist rales. If a patient has respiratory alkalosis or is compensating for metabolic acidosis, they may have deep, very fast respirations; conversely in respiratory acidosis or metabolic alkalosis compensation, their respirations are slow and shallow.
- Lastly, **blood pressure** is directly related to fluid volume levels.

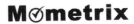

URINE VOLUME AND URINE CONCENTRATION

Both **urine volume** and **urine concentration** indicate whether a patient is experiencing homeostasis, or a state of equilibrium. Both measurements are utilized to determine whether the renal and endocrine systems are operating correctly:

- **Urine volume** is an indication of total fluid output for an individual, and it can tell the health care provider whether the patient has a total fluid volume excess or depletion.
- The **urine concentration** can point to fluid imbalances as well, because if an individual has more concentrated urine, they usually have low fluid levels as well. On the other hand, when a person has more dilute urine, they probably have a fluid volume excess in addition.

TURGOR

Turgor is a measurement of the rigidity of living cells. For human beings, tissue turgor is generally evaluated by pinching the skin and then observing the results after its release. In healthy individuals, the skin will very quickly resume its normal position, but if there is a fluid volume deficit then the skin will remain slightly elevated for a short period. In infants, skin turgor is usually observed in the abdominal area or on the thigh. On adults, the best sites to evaluate turgor are the forehead and the sternum, but the forearm or back of the hand are sometimes used as well. In older adults, turgor measurements may not be as useful because their skin is not very elastic. Tongue turgor is useful to observe as well because the presence of more than one longitudinal furrow can indicate fluid volume depletion and swelling and redness can point to sodium excess.

IMPORTANCE OF DOCUMENTING WEIGHT LOSS OR GAIN

When an individual gains or losses one kilogram of **body weight**, they have gained or lost one liter of fluid. Weight loss in a patient, while it could be an indication of tissue loss due to malnutrition or receiving supplements, is more likely to be associated with fluid loss. Rapid loss of 8% or more of body weight is generally a severe fluid volume deficiency. Sometimes, the patient may still have a fluid volume deficiency even if they do not lose weight if the fluid is retained in some other body cavity. Rapid weight gain can represent an increase in fluid volume, which can indicate retention in a variety of fluid compartments. The health care worker should measure the patient's weight every day, preferably in the morning after they void and before they eat.

OSMOLALITY

Osmolality is a measurement of the concentration of substances in a solvent, which is normally a liquid. In humans, the solvents we consider are either the serum or urine. Serum osmolality is often determined by the sodium content. It is an important measurement because if a patient is dehydrated, hyperglycemic, or has high blood urine nitrogen, they commonly have increased serum osmolality as well; conversely, with fluid volume excess, the serum osmolality is depressed. A similar concentration measurement is the urine osmolality, which is usually measured along with the serum osmolality to give a more accurate indication of the ability of the kidney to concentrate solutions. Urine specific gravity is a related test that might be also be used.

HEMATOCRIT TEST

The **hematocrit test** measures the proportion of a plasma sample that is actually comprised of red blood cells (RBCs). This is accomplished by centrifuging the sample. Males generally have 44% to 52% RBCs while females may have a slightly lower percentage, from 39% to 47%. If there is a fluid volume increase, it may be reflected in the hematocrit test with a lower percentage of red blood cells. Conversely, if a patient is dehydrated, they will have an increased hematocrit level because less fluid is present.

BUN

BUN is an abbreviation for **blood urea nitrogen**, which is basically the amount of urea present in the serum. Urea is the terminal product of the metabolism of protein. It is produced in the liver, then transferred to the circulating blood, and ultimately it is excreted by the kidneys. If a patient is overhydrated or does not ingest enough protein, they can have a low BUN. Dehydration or excessive protein intake can elevate the BUN level, which can also occur with any conditions that deplete fluids. A normal adult BUN level is between 10 and 20 mg/dL.

CAUSES OF FLUID VOLUME DEFICIT

Fluid volume deficit, or hypovolemia, can be caused by either excessive fluid loss or a diminished fluid intake:

- Abnormal **fluid loss** most commonly occurs through the gastrointestinal tract, such as when vomiting or diarrhea occurs. Fluid can also be lost through the skin, either as a means of dispelling heat when the patient's temperature is elevated, as a result of breaks in the skin, or simply as a way to control body temperature. If a hemorrhage has occurred, fluid volume can decrease in the intravascular space. Fluid can drift to areas where it cannot be utilized, such as can occur with ascites production, internal bleeding, or fluid being trapped in the bowel or other spaces.
- Hypovolemia can also occur if fluid **intake is decreased** because of inadequate intravenous solutions, lack of thirst, or inability to obtain proper fluids.

HYPERVOLEMIA

Hypervolemia is too much fluid in the extracellular compartments. Possible causes include the following:

- One of the chief causes of hypervolemia is the **intake of a surplus of sodium** and subsequent water retention. This excess sodium may come from sodium-containing intravenous solutions, sodium-rich foods or oral or IV medications that have sodium in them.
- Hypervolemia may also be caused by water or sodium retention due to **antidiuretic hormone (ADH) or aldosterone** production after surgery, or the product of other diseases, renin production, or use of corticosteroids. Fluid may be moved from the interstitial to the vascular space during burn treatment or use of certain IV solutions or medications with high osmolarity.
- There are instances as well where **individuals cannot void properly** such as in renal disease, which can lead to hypervolemia.

EDEMA

Edema is a buildup of fluid in the spaces between groups of organs or between cells, commonly called the interstitial space. Edema can occur as a consequence of inflammation. Generalized edema can also result when the patient experiences excessive sodium and water retention, or when the dynamics of exchange in their capillaries have been altered. Edema is often observed in the feet and ankles, but it can also be common in the back and buttocks if the patient has been bedridden. Severity of the edema can be assessed by measuring the area with a tape measure every day.

DIABETES

Diabetes is a disorder that causes the body to excrete excess urine:

- One form, **diabetes insipidus**, is primarily related to a water imbalance. This water imbalance is a result of a lack of antidiuretic hormone (ADH) being produced by the hypothalamus or the failure of the renal system to respond to this ADH. This condition can also be caused by head injury or metastases.
- **Diabetes mellitus**, on the other hand, results when enough insulin is not secreted or utilized. The patient typically becomes hyperglycemic with elevated blood or urine glucose levels and has ketoacidosis. They can also have depressed serum carbon dioxide levels, hypovolemia, or low potassium levels.

RESTORING FLUID AND ELECTROLYTE BALANCE AFTER BURNS

Fluid and electrolytes escape through the injured skin areas after an individual is **burned**. For about the first day, water, electrolytes and even proteins in the blood vessels are lost via the damaged capillaries and cells and edema results. Then the capillary walls begin to close back up. Several days after the burn incident, the fluid in the swollen areas begins to move into the blood vessels and consequently the blood volume increases. As a result, there is an increase in the urinary output at that point as well. Typically, intravenous fluids are also administered to burn patients to replace fluids and electrolytes.

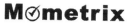

Electrolyte Disorders

ACID-BASE BALANCE

All body fluids, tissues and the bones contain chemical buffers to maintain equilibrium between acids and bases. Simply stated, an **acid** is a substance that gives up a hydrogen ion, and a **base** is one that accepts these hydrogen ions. Extracellularly the primary buffering system is bicarbonate-carbonic acid. On the other hand, there are a number of intracellular buffers. Acid-base balance is measured by examining the arterial blood gasses (ABGs).

The **four common measurements of the ABGs** include:

- **pH,** which quantifies the hydrogen ion H+ concentration.
- Partial pressure of carbon dioxide or CO_2 in the arteries or $PaCO_2$.
- Bicarbonate HCO_3 concentration.
- Partial pressure of oxygen or PaO_2 in the arteries.

METABOLIC ACIDOSIS

When the presence of metabolic acids is greater than the **concentration of bicarbonate, a low pH (below 7.35)** and **metabolic acidosis** exists. The most common causes of metabolic acidosis are diarrhea or renal excretion, with concomitant loss of bicarbonate, or increased production or ingestion of acids. This imbalance has a number of common cardiopulmonary symptoms, most notably deep and rapid respirations, a decrease in blood pressure, and dilation of the blood vessels. Low arterial pH levels can be life threatening which means sodium bicarbonate and potassium should be administered intravenously. Other diagnostic tools include low bicarbonate level, acidic urine, or elevated serum potassium levels.

RESPIRATORY ACIDOSIS

A state in which a patient cannot get rid of as much carbon dioxide as is being produced in the lungs is known as **respiratory acidosis**. Typically, the patient is usually unable to control the rate and depth of their respirations because they have been sedated, they have cerebral injury following cardiac shutdown, or they have some sort of respiratory disease. An **acidic serum pH plus a $PaCO_2$ level greater than 45 mmHg** provides a diagnosis. In addition, symptoms are usually related to effects on the central nervous system or indicators of increased cardiac output. Treatments targeting reduction of carbon dioxide include oxygen administration, inserting a tube into the windpipe, mechanical breathing assistance, bronchodilators, and sometimes antibiotics. Respiratory acidosis can be a chronic condition resulting from emphysema, cystic fibrosis, or asthma.

METABOLIC ALKALOSIS

Pathophysiology	Kidneys excrete more bicarbonate, so pH increases, and hypoventilation occurs to retain carbon dioxide and acid. Decreased strong acid or increased base, with compensatory CO_2 retention by lungs
Laboratory	Increased serum pH (>7.45). PCO$_2$ normal if uncompensated and increased (>45) if compensated. Increased HCO_3 (<26) Urine pH >6 if compensated.
Causes	Excessive vomiting, gastric suctioning, diuretics, potassium deficit, excessive mineralocorticoids and $NaHCO_3$ intake.
Symptoms	Neuro/muscular: dizziness, confusion, nervousness, anxiety, tremors, muscle cramping, tetany, tingling, seizures. Cardiac: Tachycardia and arrhythmias. GI: Nausea, vomiting, anorexia. Respiratory: Compensatory hypoventilation.
Treatment	Patient may respond to IV 0.9% saline (50 to 100 mL/hr.) but underlying cause must be identified and treated. Some patients may require hemodialysis.

EFFECTS OF LONG-TERM DIURETIC THERAPY ON ACID-BASE BALANCE

If a patient is given prolonged diuretic therapy with thiazides or furosemide, they can lose hydrogen ions or excrete bicarbonate. This can result in a condition called **chronic metabolic alkalosis**. The patient's **pH will be high, greater than 7.45.** The bicarbonate level in the arteries may be high, other electrolytes such as sodium, phosphorus, or potassium may be low, and the heart rate may be elevated. Common treatments include saline for volume expansion, oral or IV potassium chloride, or use of the type of diuretics that spare potassium (acetazolamide or Diamox).

RESPIRATORY ALKALOSIS

Respiratory alkalosis results from hyperventilation, during which extra CO_2 is excreted, causing a decrease in carbonic acid (H_2CO_3) concentration in the plasma. Respiratory alkalosis may be acute or chronic. Acute respiratory alkalosis is precipitated by anxiety attacks, hypoxemia, salicylate intoxication, bacteremia (Gram-negative), and incorrect ventilator settings. Chronic respiratory alkalosis may result from chronic hepatic insufficiency, cerebral tumors, and chronic hypocapnia.

Characteristics	Decreased $PaCO_2$ (< 35). Normal or decreased serum bicarbonate (HCO_3 <22) as kidneys conserve hydrogen and excrete HCO_3. Increased pH (>7.45).
Symptoms	Vasoconstriction with ↓cerebral blood flow resulting in lightheadedness, alterations in mentation, and/or unconsciousness. Numbness and tingling. Tinnitus. Tachycardia and dysrhythmias.
Treatment	Identifying and treating underlying cause. If respiratory alkalosis is related to anxiety, breathing in a paper bag may increase CO_2 level. Some people may require sedation. ABG values in respiratory acidosis: pH >7.45. $PaCO_2$ < 35 mm Hg. Decreased H_2CO_3 (<22).

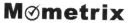

TOXEMIA OF PREGNANCY

Toxemia of pregnancy refers to a condition in pregnant women where they may be hypertensive and experience swelling or convulsions. They may also have protein in their urine. During pregnancy, fluid volume is generally enhanced, the acid-base equilibrium is typically altered, serum calcium can be depressed, and changes in renal function usually occur. A condition called **respiratory alkalosis** often results. Respiratory alkalosis is a result of excess elimination of carbon dioxide and concurrent hyperventilation. Magnesium sulfate is often given to pregnant women to prevent convulsions.

NEUROLOGICAL INDICATORS

Acid-base or electrolyte imbalances can affect **neurological parameters**. For example, electrolyte imbalances such as calcium or magnesium deficiencies can result in increased neuromuscular excitability. The excessive presence of base or metabolic alkalosis can present as tingling in the fingers or toes or dizziness. This alkalosis causes a decrease in the level of calcium ionization. Some other tests of neurological function include the Chvostek's sign where the facial nerve is pounded slightly in front of the ear to see whether the facial and eyelid muscles contract together, and the Trousseau's sign where a blood pressure cuff is inflated above the systolic pressure to see whether there the hand twitches are due to a decreased blood supply.

ELECTROLYTE SODIUM

Sodium is the major electrolyte in the extracellular fluid (ECF). It is available as a positively charged cation. Sodium levels control water distribution in the body and the volume of ECF. In the neuromuscular system, sodium increases the responsiveness of the nerve and muscle tissue and actually transmits nerve impulses. Sodium also helps to equilibrate the acid-base balance in the body. **The normal range for sodium is 135-145 mEq sodium per liter.**

HYPONATREMIA

Hyponatremia is a low level of sodium in the bodily fluids, **below 135 mEq/L.** It can be caused by too much fluid intake, either because of administration of dextrose-containing solutions, psychiatric issues, or a syndrome called SIADH. SIADH stands for syndrome of inappropriate antidiuretic hormone, where ADH is secreted unnecessarily and water retention occurs as a result. Adrenal insufficiency can also stimulate ADH. If diuretics are used or excessive sweating occurs particularly in cystic fibrosis patients, sometimes there is too much sodium loss. Symptoms include a decrease in plasma osmolality, neuromuscular effects, gastrointestinal issues, weight gain, edema, hypotension and dizziness.

HYPERNATREMIA

Hypernatremia is an excess of sodium in the bodily fluids, measured as a serum level of **greater than 145 mEq/L**. It can occur because of the presence of excess sodium or an increased loss of water. Intravenous therapy with sodium-containing solutions or medications is a typical cause of hypernatremia, but there is also a disease called primary aldosteronism, where sodium is not properly excreted. Water loss can precipitate hypernatremia as well. This loss can occur as a result of burns, sweating, impaired thirst, vapor loss from the lungs, an abnormally large urine output, or a condition called diabetes insipidus in which there is no suitable antidiuretic hormone. A patient with nervous system disorders or in a coma may have hypernatremia. They may be thirsty, have dry or sticky mucous membranes, not much saliva or tears, a rough, difficulty speaking, high temperature, or flushed skin. They can also have a low central venous pressure because of the fluid loss.

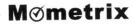

TREATMENT OF SODIUM IMBALANCES

Administration of oral or intravenous fluids is often used to **treat sodium imbalances** in a patient. If that patient is hyponatremic, hypertonic sodium chloride solutions are typically administered, but if the patient is hypernatremic solutions with low osmolality or containing 5% dextrose in water should be given. Diuretics are sometimes utilized for both conditions. In hyponatremia where there is generally a fluid excess, the diuretics help the patient to excrete this excess fluid. In patients with diabetes insipidus, they already have an increased water loss, but diuretics may still be used to lower the excessive urination that may be occur as well.

POTASSIUM

Potassium is the major positively charged electrolyte found intracellularly. Very little is found in the extracellular space, and the equilibrium between the two spaces is provided primarily through a pumping mechanism called the sodium-potassium pump. The kidneys regulate potassium levels by inducing increased excretion of potassium in the urine when serum levels are high. If potassium levels are high, more aldosterone is produced which leads to greater water and sodium retention and subsequent potassium elimination. Potassium also regulates the intracellular osmotic pressure and helps to normalize acid-base balance. **The normal range for potassium is 3.5-5.0 mEq/L.**

HYPOKALEMIA

Hypokalemia is defined as a depressed serum potassium levels, **below 3.5 mEq/L**. It can be caused by potassium loss, inadequate potassium consumption, stress, or movement of the cation into the cells. The primary cause of potassium loss is the use of diuretics and thiazides. If an individual is under stress, they may produce more aldosterone and epinephrine, which cause potassium to be either excreted or driven intracellularly. Besides common symptoms of the neuromuscular system, the most important possible symptoms of hypokalemia are related to a change in cardiac function reflected as an abnormal ECG. Blood gases usually show the patient to have a high pH, indicating they are in metabolic alkalosis.

HYPERKALEMIA

Hyperkalemia is an overly high amount of potassium in the serum **above 5.0 mEq/L.** The state is often associated with the presence of renal disease, either an acute attack or chronic. Besides increased consumption or poor potassium excretion, this condition can also be caused by the movement of potassium from inside the cells to the extracellular space by mechanisms related to metabolic acidosis and hyperglycemia. Symptoms of hyperkalemia typically involve the nerves and muscles including those of the heart. They include increased neuromuscular responses, weakness in the body and arms, and possible atrial or ventricular fibrillation and blocking of the heart. Arterial blood gases may show metabolic acidosis, and ECGs show patterns of approaching cardiac shutdown.

TREATMENT OF POTASSIUM IMBALANCES

If a patient is experiencing a potassium deficit, or hypokalemia, they may be instructed to institute dietary changes or given supplements if the case is mild. However, if levels of potassium are very low, some form intravenous potassium is usually administered. Sometimes initially the patient may be given other IV solutions just to ensure adequate hydration and kidney function.

The treatments for hyperkalemia are quite different. These include treatment with cation exchange resins, IV administration of high osmolality glucose and insulin solutions, administration of sodium bicarbonate or calcium gluconate, or dialysis. Dialysis of the blood or peritoneal fluid is used to get rid of too much potassium in extreme cases.

CALCIUM

Calcium is a positively charged electrolyte that is involved in the formation of bones and teeth, neuromuscular performance, and the clotting cascade. Calcium has an inverse relationship to phosphorus. Its production is controlled by the parathyroid hormone and calcitonin; its elimination can occur via the gastrointestinal or urinary tracts and skin as well as by bone deposition. **The normal range for serum concentration of calcium is between 8.9 and 10.3 mg/dL,** of which approximately 50% is in the ionized form and most of the rest is tied to other molecules. Only a minute percentage of the total calcium is located in the extracellular fluid.

HYPOCALCEMIA AND HYPERCALCEMIA

Since calcium concentration is regulated by the parathyroid, if this gland's regulatory functions are altered because of surgical intervention, injury, or malignancy, imbalances can occur.

- **Hypocalcemia,** defined as a serum level of **less than 4.6 mEq/L (8.9 mg/dL)** usually occurs because the intestines cannot adequately absorb the calcium or because it is lost through use of diuretics or disease or if the parathyroid glands are injured. Most symptoms of this condition are related to neuromuscular activity or respiratory effects.
- **Hypercalcemia,** defined as a serum level **above 5.1 mEq/L (10.3 mg/dL),** can be caused by increased ingestion or decreased excretion of calcium but it also can originate as a result of calcium loss from the bone itself. The latter is usually related either to hyperparathyroidism, metastatic bone disease, long periods of immobilization, or multiple fractures.

MAGNESIUM

Magnesium is a cation found mostly in the bones or muscles, and only minimally in the extracellular fluid. Magnesium plays a number of important roles in the body. These functions include activation of enzymes and regulation of protein and carbohydrate metabolism and neuromuscular regulation. In addition, magnesium can dilate blood vessels, which can affect blood pressure and cardiac output. The **normal range for serum level of magnesium is 1.3 to 2.1 mEq/L.** Low levels are associated with a variety of muscle, nerve (including mental), and cardiac abnormalities, and high levels can depress the heart rate leading to possible cardiac arrest.

PHOSPHATE

Phosphate is the primary anion found in the intracellular fluid and it is also present in the extracellular compartment. The metabolism and equilibrium concentrations of **phosphate and calcium are inversely related** and both are regulated by the parathyroid gland. Phosphate is important in the metabolism of protein, fats and carbohydrates, energy transfer, the promotion of acid-base balance, and the stimulation of muscle and nerve activity. In renal disease, it is important to look for hyperphosphatemia, or phosphate excess, because the kidney's ability to excrete phosphate is diminished. The **normal range for serum phosphate is 2.5-4.5 mg/dL.**

CHLORIDE

Chloride is the main negatively charged electrolyte found in the extracellular fluid and its level is directly related to the levels of both sodium and potassium cations. It has a reverse relationship to the amount of bicarbonate present. Chloride helps to regulate water movement. The cation also helps maintain acid-base equilibrium and the reabsorption of sodium. When IV solutions with potassium or sodium are given continuously or too much or during metabolic acidosis as an adjunct to dehydration or bicarbonate loss, excess chloride or hyperchloremia, can also result. The **normal range for chloride values are 97 to 100 mEq/L.**

Maintenance and Replacement

TONICITY

Tonicity is an ongoing energetic process whereby particles or molecules move from one compartment to another in the body. While small molecules can easily shift between compartments, larger ones cannot move as easily. The molecule size combined with the permeability of the membrane determines the rate of movement of fluids and electrolytes between compartments. Solutions can be hypotonic, isotonic or hypertonic:

- A **hypotonic solution** has a solute concentration lower than that generally found in bodily fluids, defined as less than 240 mOsm/kg.
- **Isotonic solutions** have an osmolality similar to plasma with a range of 240 to 340 mOsm/kg.
- **Hypertonic solutions** have a higher osmolality, above 340 mOsm/kg.

When a **hypotonic solution** is administered, the fluid is drawn intracellularly. This type of solution, for example 0.45% sodium chloride, is sometimes used to treat situations where there is an electrolyte excess. **Isotonic solutions**, which include 0.9% saline, 5% dextrose in water, and Lactated Ringer's, are often given to rapidly increase the extravascular volume. This is because water by itself will not generally move from one space to another. **Hypertonic solutions** add high solute concentrations, which result in greater fluid pressure. Therefore, they pull fluid out of cells and cause them to shrink, a trait making them useful to decrease intracellular fluid or for volume expansion. Hypertonic solutions include 3% or 5% sodium chloride or 50% dextrose in water.

DEXTROSE SOLUTIONS

Dextrose in water is either administered as an isotonic solution (5%) or at higher hypertonic concentrations. Since these fluids do not contain electrolytes, their main functions are to hydrate and to provide calories to the patient. Particularly in the very concentrated hypertonic solutions, 20% dextrose and above, administration is done to provide calories. Amino acids may be included as well to enhance total nutrition. 50% dextrose in water is usually utilized to counteract low blood sugar levels related to hypoglycemia. Dextrose may also be administered in solution with various hypertonic concentrations of sodium chloride. These combinations not only provide calories but can also provide needed electrolytes and provide fluid volume expansion.

RINGER'S SOLUTION

Ringer's solution or injection by itself is an isotonic solution that mimics the electrolyte composition of plasma. It contains sodium, potassium, calcium and chloride. If lactate is added as a buffer, the solution is called **Lactated Ringer's injection (Hartmann solution).** The added lactate will metabolize to produce bicarbonate, which is normally present in the extracellular fluid. Both of these variations provide fluid and electrolytes, but no calorie requirements when used alone. Furthermore, the lactated version should not be used in hepatic disorders or lactic acidosis. 5% dextrose is commonly added to both types of Ringer's solutions to provide calorie intake, but in doing so the solution becomes hypertonic. Therefore, when administering the dextrose-containing injections, one must watch for fluid volume excess or complications from diabetes mellitus.

PLASMA EXPANDERS

Plasma expanders are colloidal solutions given in order to expand the intravascular compartments, usually administered in emergency situations. They can include blood components, the innate plasma protein albumin, or synthetic colloids. The commonly given synthetic colloids are dextran, mannitol, and hetastarch (Hespan). Dextran solutions can contain either high or low

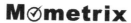

molecular weight dextran commonly diluted into either 5% dextrose or 0.9% saline. In either case, the main use for dextran solutions is restoration of vascular volume that has been depressed due to some traumatic event. The health care provider must watch for possible hypersensitivity to dextran and subsequent anaphylactic reactions. Mannitol is a sugar alcohol, found commercially in solutions from 5% to 25%; it is primarily used to stimulate loss of fluid thereby decreasing pressure. Hespan, found in 6% concentration in 0.9% saline, is similar in use and complications to dextran. Albumin is normally administered during shock to promote volume expansion.

Mechanisms Involved for Unique Solutions Administered to Maintain Fluid and Electrolyte Balance

Solutions with a high or alkaline pH, most commonly 5% sodium bicarbonate, might be given to a patient in order to normalize excess acids. This is accomplished by dissociation of the compound to generate bicarbonate anion, which is the major buffer in the extracellular fluid. A hypertonic alcohol solution, typically 5% ethyl alcohol in 5% dextrose might be administered as a substitute for water with the addition of calories. The mechanism here is metabolism of the ethyl alcohol in the liver into acetaldehyde or acetate. There are also a variety of premixed IV solutions available that can be beneficial because they either include medications or provide the appropriate buffering capacity or pH.

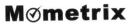

Parenteral Nutrition

TYPES OF PARENTERAL NUTRITION

Parenteral nutrition is the process of providing either partial or total nutrient requirements to a patient via the venous system. There are two main types, either peripheral parenteral nutrition (PPN) or total parenteral nutrition (TPN):

- **PPN** provides only some nutritional requirements and should only be used for a short while or as supplemental support. It involves infusing a low osmolarity solution of dextrose, electrolytes, amino acids, vitamins, fat and trace elements by using peripheral veins.
- **TPN** introduces higher concentrations of these components using a central vein and provides complete nutrition.

Parenteral nutrition should only be used when oral or enteral routes cannot be utilized because if the gastrointestinal tract is resting, adverse side effects can occur. The time to consider starting parenteral nutrition is generally after 5 to 7 days after a patient has been unable to eat normally.

TPN

TPN provides nutrition via a central vein and is riskier than PPN, but TPN also supplies greater nutritional needs without introducing large fluid volumes. TPN is utilized as the primary therapy for the gastrointestinal tract diseases short gut syndrome and enterocutaneous fistula. It is also provided in cases of allogeneic bone transplantation, acute Crohn's disease, severe necrotizing pancreatitis, and uncontrollable nausea with vomiting. The use of TPN for diseases such as anorexia nervosa and inflammatory disease has not been proven but is common practice. Sometimes, total parenteral nutrition is employed as an adjunct for cancer patients, when septicemia is present, or during surgery or some other type of trauma. Disorders of the gastrointestinal tract and sometimes the respiratory tract indicate use of TPN in pediatric patients.

TOTAL DAILY ENERGY EXPENDITURE

An individual's **total daily energy (TDE) expenditure** is mixture of a number of components, and they all need to be considered to determine nutritional requirements. The largest component, accounting for up to about three-quarters of energy expenditure, is the basal energy expenditure (BEE), also called BMR. This is the base energy expenditure rate and can be estimated using formulas relating to weight, height, age and gender. A simpler estimation of BEE is 30 to 35 calories per kg of weight. The most accurate method to determine caloric requirements is indirect calorimetry which measures oxygen consumption and carbon dioxide production. The other components to total daily energy expenditure are activity level and the specific dynamic action (SDA) of food referring to the increased heat production that occurs during eating or receiving infusions.

MALNUTRITION

A patient is considered **malnourished** or **at risk** if they do not have adequate nutrient intake for a week or more or if they lose at least 10% of their body weight. This condition is primarily due to a lack of either protein or total caloric intake. There are three classifications of malnutrition. The first, marasmus, is a chronic condition where there is a slow wasting of the fat just below the skin (adipose) and somatic muscle occurs but the visceral proteins are still intact; its genesis is a reduced total dietary intake such as in starvation, anorexia, chronic illness or aging. Kwashiorkor, or hypoalbuminemia, can present when the diet is overwhelmingly carbohydrate in nature with little or no protein intake such as with liquid diets or use of IV dextrose solutions. In this case, the visceral protein stores are depleted and extracellular spaces fill up with water. A combination of the

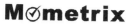

two, marasmus-kwashiorkor, sometimes occurs in hospitalized patients with pre-existing marasmus who are then treated with IV dextrose solutions. All of these can impair the immune system.

DISEASES THAT AFFECT NUTRITIONAL STATUS
DISEASES OF THE ESOPHAGUS, STOMACH, OR INTESTINE

Sometimes the ingestion of nutrients is immediately inhibited in the **esophagus** by an obstruction or the inability to pass the food. The **stomach** can be dysfunctional whereby food either cannot be ingested or passed onto the small intestine. Diseases such as a peptic ulcer or gastric cancer can cause these malfunctions, but in addition a mechanical obstruction or surgery may precipitate specific incidents such as delayed emptying or a rapid discharge (dumping syndrome). **Intestinal diseases** are more common and include short bowel syndrome, a postoperative syndrome characterized by intense diarrhea and loss of fluid and electrolytes followed by subsequent ability to stabilize and adapt; inflammatory bowel disease (Crohn's disease or ulcerative colitis) caused by decreased intake, increased output, or malabsorption; and pancreatitis, where patients usually cannot metabolize carbohydrates or absorb nutrients and have weight loss and other issues.

DISEASES OF THE LIVER AND GALLBLADDER DISEASES

The **liver** is a metabolic storage vehicle. In other words, a variety of metabolic processes occur there including protein synthesis, the elimination of the bile, metabolism of toxins and nutrient regulation. If the liver is impaired such as in hepatitis or cirrhosis of the liver, untoward metabolic changes occur such as glucose or protein intolerance or their synthesis, altered ability to process fats, an increased requirement for nitrogen, and impaired storage of trace elements. Dietary intake is impaired from loss through nausea and vomiting but also because of psychological problems or alcohol use. Cholecystitis, inflammation of the **gallbladder** as a result of infection or postoperative stress, can lead to poor intake or increased loss of nutrients as well. If there is a biliary tract obstruction, poor eating habits or increased protein and caloric requirements may occur. A condition called steatorrhea, or excess fat in the stools, can result because fats and fat-soluble vitamins are not absorbed.

PHYSIOLOGICAL DIFFERENCES AND NUTRIENT IMBALANCES IN ACUTE AND CHRONIC RENAL FAILURE

Chronic renal failure usually occurs secondarily to a number of a number of other mouth or gastrointestinal conditions. These types of conditions lead to a wasting of the lean body tissue and muscle mass and concomitant fluid retention as well as increased nutrient requirements. Acute renal failure results from a number of the same conditions or as a precedent to a comatose situation. In this case, the acute episode may be precipitated by the buildup of toxic protein metabolites and electrolyte imbalance as a result of the severe breakdown of endogenous proteins.

BODILY CHANGES IN DIABETES MELLITUS THAT AFFECT NUTRITIONAL STATUS

An individual with **diabetes mellitus** has difficulty properly taking in and metabolizing mainly carbohydrates but other nutritional needs are affected as well. A hallmark of diabetes mellitus is that highly elevated plasma glucose levels or increased blood sugars are observed which leads to glucose in the urine and osmotic diuresis. If glucose is infused, the patient has difficulty oxidizing it. Fat metabolism is affected as well with increased lysis of lipids, fat oxidation and glycerol turnover. There is a net protein catabolism either through increased breakdown or decreased synthesis.

COPD AND MALNUTRITION

In patients with **chronic obstructive pulmonary disease, or COPD,** severe weight loss often occurs. An individual with COPD expends quite a bit of energy as well during their labored breathing plus at times they have an oxygen deficit which affects metabolism. This can lead to malnutrition, which for these patients is defined as being less than 90% of ideal body weight or losing more 15% of their weight. Weight loss sometimes approaches a quarter of their body weight. Another respiratory condition, acute respiratory distress syndrome, can occur in individuals taking bronchodilators or other drugs. In this condition, oxygen transport is depressed secondarily to low phosphate levels.

CANCER CACHEXIA

Chronic diseases can sometimes cause **cachexia** which is general physical and mental debilitation caused by weakness and appetite loss. Cancer patients often experience a form of it called cancer cachexia not only because of the tumor itself but because of the chemotherapy treatments they are receiving or they are depressed. Anorexia and severe malnutrition are common in these patients and a number of metabolic abnormalities develop. Protein levels are depleted through increased turnover, lipid reserves are depleted, and insulin resistance often develops.

EFFECTS OF STRESS, TRAUMA OR BURNS ON THE METABOLIC PROCESS

Stress, trauma or burns are all traumatic events that in general increase metabolism. Critically ill patients in particular often experience stress which can in turn create severe nutritional defects. The main reason for this is more cytokines are produced; cytokines are proteins which affect the metabolism of cells. In trauma, these metabolic alterations occur from the time of the incident until the completion of wound healing and recovery. After a burn injury, pathophysiologic changes are found to a large extent in the gastrointestinal tract and a condition called ileus, an incapacity of the intestine to pass its contents, can result. If the injury is severe, there is increased metabolism and nitrogen loss as well as greater energy consumption.

SIGNS OF NUTRITIONAL DEFICIENCIES

Signs of nutritional deficiencies are most commonly observed visually in the skin, hair, eyes or mouth of the patient being assessed by the health care provider. This is especially true for the skin, an area that can reveal a number of nutritional deficiencies. The individual may be deficient in vitamin A or essential fatty acids if their skin is dry or flaky or they present with follicular hyperkeratosis. If they have petechiae, vitamins C or K may be lacking. Niacin deficiency may be present if the individual has increased pigmentation on body parts with sun exposure, known as pellagrous dermatosis. If patients are malnourished, their hair can be dull and thinning or changing colors or they might have hair loss. Examination of the nails can reveal an iron deficiency. Patients with nutritional defects may have purple or very red tongues, mouth tears (due to B vitamins), shrunken taste buds, patchy teeth enamel (due to fluorine excess), or bleeding gums (associated with vitamin C deficiency).

ANTHROPOMETRIC MEASUREMENTS

Anthropometric measurements are physical evaluations of subcutaneous fat and muscle mass. The latter is in theory indicative of the somatic protein levels. However, these measurements can be unreliable because the measurements can be inflated by presence of swelling and or indeterminate because of inconsistencies of measurement. Height and weight would be considered anthropometric measurements as well but again the latter is more useful when done as a series of measurements. There is also another test called the **creatinine-height index (CHI)**, which measures creatinine excretion in the urine. Theoretically, the amount of creatinine is proportional to the skeletal muscle mass but again inconsistencies in collection or dietary intake and renal disease can all affect results.

94

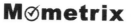

LABORATORY TESTS FOR MALNUTRITION

Serum albumin is often used to assess the possibility of malnutrition because albumin is by far the most prevalent protein in the body, up to 65%, and it acts as a carrier protein. Albumin is synthesized in the liver and it also has a long half-life, 18 days. Therefore, its usefulness as an indicator of malnourishment or recovery is limited because low levels might be due to liver function or fluid changes instead or changes happen too slowly to measure accurately. Serum **transferrin** and **prealbumin** are also used as tests for levels of visceral protein. They are carrier proteins for iron and retinol-binding proteins respectively. Both proteins have shorter half-lives than albumin as well, 8 days for transferrin and one to two days for prealbumin. The **retinol-binding protein** itself is sometimes measured too, but its usefulness is limited because it has a very short half-life, 18 hours at most.

IMMUNOLOGICAL TESTS TO ASSESS MALNUTRITION

Nutritional deficiencies as well as stress or disease states can affect immunocompetency. The two commonly utilized **immunological tests** to determine nutritional status are total lymphocyte count and delayed cutaneous hypersensitivity or anergy testing. A total **lymphocyte count** is a measurement derived from a routine differential blood count:

$$Total\ lymphocyte\ count = (\%\ lymphocytes\ x\ white\ blood\ count)/100$$

Levels less than 1200/mm³ suggests malnutrition. In **delayed cutaneous hypersensitivity testing**, a panel of four or more typical skin test antigens is injected into the skin. This injection should elicit a local inflammatory response within 48 to 72 hours to at least some of the antigens if the T lymphocytes are working properly. Anergy, the absence of response to any of these antigens, may indicate severe malnutrition.

MEASURING NITROGEN BALANCE

Measurements of nitrogen balance represent the difference between nitrogen intake and output through excretion and other means. They are done to look at baseline nutritional status and then to follow the progress of nutritional support. The net nitrogen balance is directly related to the net in protein. Nitrogen intake is calculated as the protein intake divided by 6.25. Output is determined from urea nitrogen output plus estimations of other losses such as insensible and gastrointestinal. Nutrients should be increased if the expected positive nitrogen balance is not achieved.

CYCLIC AND CONTINUOUS SOLUTION ADMINISTRATION REGIMENS

TPN is usually administered **continuously** initially, starting at a rate of 60 to 80 mL/hr for the first day and then increasing the rate at 20mL/hr increments every day or two. If the patient is stable or receiving therapy at home, the continuous TPN can be transitioned to cyclic administration. **Cyclic administration** typically involves cycling the infusion in 8- to 16-hour blocks of time. The hourly rate still needs to accommodate the desired daily needs of the patients so it may be greater than continuous administration. Cyclic administration must be initiated gradually and is usually done at night. Complications can include compromised cardiovascular status due to fluid overload, increased possibility of infection, and hyperglycemia.

PRECAUTIONS BEFORE INFUSING LIPIDS

Before infusing **lipids**, bring the emulsion to room temperature because cold solutions cause paling of the skin and pain. Inspect the solution for foaming, signs of layering, or an oily appearance. Normal filtration cannot be done because the lipids will clog the filter and the emulsion could separate, but a 1.2-micron filter might be utilized for three-in-one preparations. Start with a test dose to observe any possible adverse reactions; a typical test dose would be infusion for up to a half

95

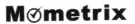

hour. Then, the regular infusion might be done over a period of 4 to 6 hours for 10% solutions, 6 to 8 hours for 20% solutions.

SELF-MONITORING FOR HOME PARENTERAL NUTRITION

Some patients require extended or even permanent intravenous feeding and are sent home with either percutaneously placed catheters (if short-term up to 3 months) or long-term tunneled catheters or implanted ports. They are then instructed in self or family-aided infusion, usually done on a cyclic basis. These individuals need to be instructed on a number of issues including symptoms that they can monitor themselves every day, such as fever, chills, swelling, and weight changes that are sudden or outside the expected parameters. They need to be instructed on how to monitor their fluid consumed and their urinary excretion because ideally their total output should be about a half liter less than that consumed; if they excrete excessive amounts, they are probably receiving too much fluid. Of course, instructions on handling of emergencies are essential.

PARENTERAL NUTRITION FORMULAS

PPN formulas for peripheral nutrition usually contain lower concentrations of dextrose and amino acids than other types. A typical PPN formula contains 1.75% to 3.5% amino acids and 5% to 10% dextrose, as well as up to 20% lipids. TPN formulations generally contain 4.25% amino acids and 25% dextrose along with electrolytes, trace elements and vitamins. Three-in-one solutions usually up the amino acids to 5% while lowering the dextrose concentration to 17.5% and adding a 10% lipid suspension. Formulations intended for infants or young children often contain amino acids that are essential for that age group but not adults.

AMINO ACIDS AND DIETARY PROTEIN

Protein is utilized in the body to help promote tissue growth and repair and to replace of all of the cells in the body. It is found in either somatic tissues such as the skeletal muscle and the skeleton or in the viscera as solid viscera or secretory proteins. Protein is always being turned over in the body, and its components, the amino acids, are released, ultimately producing nitrogen which is excreted in the urine as urea. The only place amino acids are stored is in muscle mass and therefore they must be constantly replaced, usually via ingestion of protein. One goal of total parenteral nutrition, therefore, is to maintain nitrogen equilibrium.

FORMULATION AND CALORIC VALUE OF PROTEIN IN PARENTERAL NUTRITION

The three essential nutrients commonly included in parenteral nutrition formulations are carbohydrates, fats and proteins **because** each contributes to protein buildup and tissue synthesis. Protein solutions are usually available as crystalline amino acids in concentrations ranging up to 15% with or without addition of electrolytes. Special branched-chained amino acids are also sold and sometimes used in hepatic and renal diseases or during stress or sepsis. Amino acid solutions represent a caloric value of 4.0 calories per gram, but with addition of other nutrients in total parenteral nutrition the maximum amount that can be infused is about 180 grams a day.

CARBOHYDRATES IN PARENTERAL NUTRITION

Carbohydrates provide approximately half of the calories and energy in life. For nutritional solutions, a carbohydrate source is usually supplied for the same purpose, most often in the form of dextrose (glucose) which is a physiologic substrate. Other sources sometimes used are fructose, sorbitol, xylitol, and glycerol. Fructose, a naturally occurring monosaccharide as well as the alcohol sugars sorbitol and xylitol all must be converted to glucose in the liver before they can be utilized. Glycerol has not been well studied. If glucose is given as a nutrient, any not immediately utilized to provide energy is stored in the liver and muscle as glycogen or fat if there is not enough capacity.

96

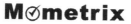

INTRAVENOUS ADMINISTRATION OF FAT

Fats provide at least double the amount of energy on a calorie per gram basis as either protein or carbohydrates, and they can be introduced into peripheral veins because they are isotonic. The benefits of fat or lipid infusions include the avoidance of complications resulting from large glucose intake as well as reduction of fat deposition in the liver and lower levels of circulating insulin. Fats in the form of triglycerides, phospholipids, cholesterol or fatty acids perform a large range of metabolic and structural functions. Intravenous administration of fats can deter a condition called essential fatty acid deficiency (EFAD) which causes symptoms ranging from hemolytic anemia to hepatic malfunction. Up to 60% of calories can be infused as lipid.

EFFECTS OF PARENTERAL NUTRITION ON ELECTROLYTES OR ESSENTIAL MACRONUTRIENTS

Electrolytes could be considered essential macronutrients. If a patient has is malnourished, he loses the electrolytes needed to retain nitrogen while developing an excess of sodium and water. The ability to retain nitrogen needs to be restored via administration of the potassium or magnesium cations some form of phosphorus without fluid or sodium overload. Chloride levels must approximate sodium levels, which is often accomplished with use of acetate-containing amino acid formulations. During refeeding of malnourished individuals, phosphate can be redistributed into the muscle causing hypophosphatemia. Serum calcium levels are often low in the malnourished and need replacement. Gastrointestinal secretion of magnesium may require its inclusion as well.

TRACE ELEMENTS

The following **trace elements** are found in the body and may be included with nutritional supplementation:

- **Iron:** Involved in oxygen transport, occasionally added as iron dextran.
- **Iodine:** Used to produce thyroid hormone.
- **Zinc:** Found in many enzymes and cofactors and necessary for synthesis of RNA, DNA and protein.
- **Copper:** Used for normal production of red blood cells as well as part of oxidative enzymes.
- **Chromium:** Increases the effectiveness of insulin binding to tissue receptors.
- **Manganese:** Numerous functions including antioxidant, enzymatic cofactor, involved in connective tissue formation and carbohydrate synthesis from pyruvate.
- **Selenium:** Catalyzes glutathione peroxidase in the antioxidant pathway.
- **Molybdenum:** Sulfite oxidase and xanthine oxidase cofactor.

VITAMINS

Vitamins are organic compounds required for normal growth and support of body functions because they serve as cofactors with a number of enzymes. They must be supplemented in the diet because they cannot be adequately synthesized in the body. Some vitamins are **fat-soluble**, including vitamins A, D, E and K. All the others are **water-soluble**, including things like thiamine, vitamin B_{12}, pantothenic acid, and ascorbic acid or Vitamin C. The solubility determines the type of solution if administered as an infusion, which is definitely different from oral administration, because the gut and liver cannot play the same role of modifying and storing the vitamin as they do when ingested.

FAT-SOLUBLE VITAMINS

The 4 **fat-soluble vitamins** are:

- **Vitamin A:** Keeps epithelial surfaces intact, protects against disease, and aids synthesis of retinal pigments; lack can cause various sight problems.
- **Vitamin D**: Aids calcium and phosphate absorption and mobilizes calcium from the bone; deficiency associated with bone deformities and muscle pain and spasms.
- **Vitamin E**: Tissue antioxidant; if low, primarily blood abnormalities can occur.
- **Vitamin K**: Necessary for synthesis of clotting factors II, VII, IX and X; deficiency can cause bleeding and associated symptoms.

WATER-SOLUBLE VITAMINS

Water-soluble vitamins are as follows:

- **Thiamine (B1)**: Part of cocarboxylase enzyme complex, an energy source; muscle or neural defects can be a result of deficiency.
- **Riboflavin (B2)**: Coenzyme to lipoproteins that promote tissue oxidation and respiration; if low, oral and visual disturbances can be observed.
- **Niacin**: Part of coenzymes for nicotinamide compounds required for glycolysis, fat synthesis, and energy creation; dermatitis, diarrhea, neural disorders, anorexia can result from deficiency.
- **Pantothenic acid**: A portion of coenzyme A, which helps production of energy from carbohydrate synthesis of fats; symptoms of deficiency include abdominal issues, headache and lethargy.
- **Pyridoxine (B6)**: Amino acid metabolic cofactor, involved with neurotransmitters and in heme protein synthesis; if deficient, can see central nervous system abnormalities, inflamed tongue, anemia.
- **Biotin (B7)**: Enzyme cofactor in multiple systems; skin rash, neural and muscular disturbances, anemia, anorexia, and more could be caused by deficiency.
- **Folacin (folic acid)**: Transfers carbon units as tetrahydrofolate; if lack, can see anemia, malabsorption, stomatitis and more.
- **Vitamin B12**: Involved with nucleic acid formation; if deficient, can see anemia, inflammation, neuropathy.
- **Ascorbic acid (vitamin C)**: Has a wide range of roles in growth, amino acid hydroxylation, gastrointestinal absorption, etc.; deficiency slows down wound healing and can cause gingivitis and scurvy.

DEXTROSE

Dextrose or **glucose** is by far the most widely used source of carbohydrates in parenteral solutions. Generally, it is well tolerated and can be given in large amounts. Daily caloric needs can be met with carbohydrates alone, although lipids are often included to enhance nitrogen balance or tissue production. Dextrose provides 3.4 calories per gram. Precautionary measures are needed, however, because infusing excessive amounts of glucose can cause hyperglycemia, increased production and storage of fat, liver malfunction, or respiratory failure due to excessive carbon dioxide production.

LIPID EMULSIONS

Commercially available **lipid emulsions** are dispersions in water of a neutral triglyceride, typically an oil, to which other lipids may be added such as egg yolk phospholipid as a suspension agent or glycerol to make the solution isotonic. The lipids are a caloric source and also can treat essential fatty acid deficiency. These long-chain fatty acids are a great source of the essential fatty acid called linoleic acid. Caloric value is 1.1 or 2.0 calories/mL for the 10% and 20% formulations respectively. Formulations are available as 10% or 20% concentrations in isotonic solution and can be given either peripherally or centrally. Possible adverse effects include impaired immune responses including anaphylaxis, fever, back or chest pain, cyanosis, headache, and gastrointestinal issues. The clinician needs to watch for short-term changes in liver function, blood coagulation or cholesterol levels.

ADDING INSULIN, HEPARIN, OR HISTAMINE ANTAGONISTS TO NUTRITION FOR INFUSION

Insulin is thought to be chemically stable when added to parenteral nutrition solutions. Addition of regular insulin (not other forms) to these solutions generally does not cause hypoglycemia because of its rapid turnover. Some patients need the insulin to maintain normal blood glucose levels during administration of glucose solutions. Another use of insulin would be IV or subcutaneous administration to manage hyperglycemic attacks. **Heparin** is sometimes added to nutritional solutions to prevent formation of a fibrin sleeve and subsequent thrombosis. **Histamine antagonists** might be included to inhibit gastric acid secretion often as a prophylactic device against stress-induced ulcers.

TOTAL NUTRIENT ADMIXTURE

A **total nutrient admixture**, sometimes called a "three-in-one," is a nutritional solution which has lipids already mixed in with other components, typically amino acids, carbohydrates, electrolytes, and trace elements. Usually lipids are given as a unique infusion, but including the "three-in-one" formulation decreases the quantity of calories from glucose and thus is particularly useful in diabetic patients or those with suppressed respiratory function. The issue of possible microbial infection is two-sided with these formulations, because although they require fewer manipulations of the administration set, they also cannot be filtered through a 0.2-micron filter to capture bacteria. Risk of infection with *Staphylococcus epidermidis, Candida albicans,* and *Escherichia coli* exists. The admixing of all these reagents can result in precipitates, and the lipid particles can aggregate.

MANIPULATION OF NUTRITIONAL FORMULATIONS TO TREAT SPECIFIC DISEASES

Disease-specific nutritional formulations are often employed for infusion in patients experiencing renal failure, hepatic failure or some type of stress. The changes are generally in the use of different or additional amino acids. In renal failure, patients undergo dialysis which depletes both essential and nonessential amino acids. Therefore, normally nonessential amino acids, notably histidine, are added to high levels of essential amino acids in the solution. Individuals with hepatic failure typically have increased amounts of aromatic amino acids and low concentrations of branched-chain amino acids (BCAAs), so the formulations used may be low in aromatic and high in BCAAs. Patients under stress may exhibit a similar pattern of amino acid distribution and may be given similar formulations.

TECHNICAL OR SEPTIC COMPLICATIONS WITH PARENTERAL NUTRITIONAL ADMINISTRATION

When peripheral catheters are inserted, phlebitis or thrombophlebitis can occur because of high osmolarity, low pH or presence of particles. This can be diminished by adding heparin, hydrocortisone or sodium bicarbonate or the simultaneous infusion of lipid emulsions to act as buffers and decrease the concentration of dextrose. Infection or sepsis can be observed with nutritional infusions but this is primarily found with three-in-one solutions or lipid emulsions, because the lipid provides a growth substrate for gram-positive or gram-negative bacteria or fungi.

Normally TPN solutions have several bacteriostatic components. Septicemia is prevalent in patients receiving TPN primarily because their disease states and interventions are so complex.

COMPLICATIONS FROM PARENTERAL NUTRITION

ESSENTIAL FATTY ACID DEFICIENCY AND VITAMIN DEFICIENCY

Parenteral nutrition is the provision of fluid and nutrients intravenously in order to prevent malnutrition in patients who are not able to obtain nutrition through the digestive system. Complications may include:

- **Essential fatty acid deficiency**: With deficiency, the patient may experience dry flaky skin and thrombocytopenia. Management is by increasing lipid intake with lipids added to TPN solution at least twice weekly, oral fats if tolerated, and application of topical fats to the skin to prevent tissue breakdown.
- **Vitamin deficiency**: Multivitamin preparations contain 100% of recommended daily requirements for all vitamins, so vitamin levels in TPN solution are usually sufficient although many patients may already have vitamin D or other deficiency and may need supplementation. Individual vitamin levels should be assessed periodically and vitamin intake increased if necessary. Patients receiving warfarin should have vitamin K levels monitored.

TRACE MINERAL DEFICIENCY

The **signs and symptoms** of trace mineral deficiency:

- **Chromium**: Hyperlipidemia, glucose intolerance, neuropathy.
- **Copper**: Peripheral numbness, weakness, ataxia, leukopenia, anemia (hypochromatic, microcytic, normocytic).
- **Manganese**: Weight loss, dermatitis.
- **Selenium**: Depigmentation, muscle soreness/myopathy, cardiomyopathy, anemia (macrocytic).
- **Zinc**: Dermatitis, hair loss, anorexia, immunocompromise, stomatitis, glossitis, depressed healing.

The **management** of trace mineral deficiency:

Trace element additions to parenteral nutrition formulas are based on weight. If deficiency is noted, care must be taken to avoid toxic doses. Some elements are generally found in TPN formulas: chromium, copper, manganese, molybdenum, selenium, and zinc.

Monitoring of trace elements can be problematical, so additions are usually based on clinical findings and other tests, such as glucose response (chromium), whole blood manganese test, erythrocyte glutathione peroxidase activity (selenium), and ceruloplasmin (copper).

REFEEDING SYNDROME

Refeeding syndrome refers to the cardiac abnormalities that may initially occur when extremely malnourished individuals are begun on nutritional infusion therapy. If someone is severely malnourished, they will often have depleted cardiac reserves and they will be primarily using stored body fat for metabolism. When parenteral nutrition is begun, the primary source for metabolic processes shifts from fats to carbohydrates. If the therapy is not begun slowly, severe imbalances can occur. The most common symptoms of this syndrome, therefore, are cardiac in

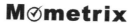

nature including among others hypercapnia, which is elevated blood levels of CO_2, and possible cardiac arrest.

ELECTROLYTE BALANCES THAT CAN OCCUR WITH NUTRITIONAL THERAPY

The plasma levels of the electrolytes **phosphorus, potassium, or magnesium** may fall during initial stages of nutritional therapy. In the case of phosphorus, this occurs because as the TPN is infused the phosphate is redistributed into the muscles, it is utilized for protein synthesis, and it is also transferred into the intracellular space as adenosine triphosphate. Both potassium and magnesium can also be shifted into the intracellular space; severe serum depletion of potassium can occur. Conversely, sodium is shifted from the intracellular to the extracellular space in order to maintain equilibrium.

HYPERGLYCEMIA OR HYPOGLYCEMIA SECONDARY TO NUTRITIONAL TREATMENT

Most TPN solutions contain high concentrations of dextrose. Therefore, individuals with diabetes or some other abnormalities who might be glucose intolerant can develop a syndrome of **hyperglycemia** and associated high osmolarity if TPN infusion is done too quickly. This happens because they cannot metabolize the glucose at that rate, which for individuals with normal insulin response is about 0.5 g/kg/hr. The first indicator of hyperglycemia is usually glucose in the urine but if it is not treated with the addition of insulin, increased urine output, coma and death can occur. Conversely, if these high glucose solutions are abruptly stopped or decreased, **hypoglycemia** can occur. The latter condition is primarily found in children.

MONITORING LIVER FUNCTION DURING TPN

Liver function abnormalities associated with hepatic complications are one of the most prevalent issues to consider with TPN. In fact, hepatic damage has been observed in about a third of infants receiving nutritional therapy and up to half of infants with low birth weights. The earliest sign of liver function abnormality portending hepatic complications is usually an elevated level of direct or conjugated bilirubin, and this is followed by other elevated hepatic enzymes. Long-term TPN has been associated with cholestasis, a condition where bile flow is stopped, and gallbladder disease. Hepatic abnormalities in infants can lead to fatality.

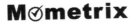

Infusion Therapy Complications

MAJOR COMPLICATIONS WHEN DRUGS ARE ADMINISTERED

Some drugs or other agents are either vesicants or irritants. Vesicants can cause blisters or destroy tissue when they leak into surrounding tissue, known as extravasation. Extravasation of irritants can produce pain in the vein at the site and sometimes inflammation. Even if the agent is not a vesicant or irritant, complications can arise if it is administered accide1ntally into the surrounding tissue. If two drugs are given simultaneously, they could affect each other either by antagonism, synergism, or potentiation. In other words, the action of one drug could cross react and be inhibited by the other, the drugs acting together could produce either unique or enhanced reactions, or in extreme cases greatly enhanced reactions occur. A patient might be allergic to the reagent and anaphylactic shock could occur after administration. Another type of shock called speed shock can happen with rapid injection. Bacterial infections or some other type of disturbance could be introduced that inflames the walls of the vein, causing a condition called phlebitis as a result.

LOCAL MECHANICAL COMPLICATIONS DURING INFUSION

Local mechanical complications of infusion therapy usually involve the insertion site, the catheter itself, the solution container, or the administration set. If swelling occurs near the site, infiltration or bleeding into the surrounding tissues has probably occurred. If a catheter has been inserted against a vessel wall or if it is kinked or bent, the flow rate can be depressed or stopped completely. These problems can be fixed by pulling or taping or removing the catheter. If a catheter has been placed near joints that bend, the flow rate may increase and decrease with flexion and extension; this can be corrected by repositioning or using an arm board. Defective catheters should be removed. Mechanical problems with the solution container can include an empty container, absence of proper gravity flow (place 30 inches above the heart), the need to air vent the container (usually a glass bottle), obstructed bag-entry ports, or use of solutions that are too cold. Pinched, crimped, or kinked administration sets or occlusion of attached filters can impede flow as well as anything acting like a tourniquet.

INFUSION-RELATED COMPLICATIONS OF ECCHYMOSIS AND HEMATOMA

When a skin area is bruised, bleeding can occur into the surrounding area; this is termed ecchymosis. **Ecchymosis** can in term develop into the formation of a **hematoma**, which is basically a semisolid mass of blood in the tissues. Symptoms are tissue discoloration from blood infiltration and swelling once the hematoma is formed. If severe, these conditions can actually limit the use of the extremity. In either case, the catheter should be removed immediately. Heavy pressure that could increase the bleeding should be avoided, and if a hematoma has developed the extremity should be elevated and ice applied to the area.

INFILTRATION

Infiltration is the accidental administration of a <u>non-vesicant</u> medication or solution into tissues adjacent to a vascular pathway instead of into the vessel itself. This complication usually occurs when a catheter is dislodged. If the health care provider observes that the skin is tight or flexion/extension is difficult, they should suspect infiltration. This condition also produces pale or cool skin and a tender site. Acidic or alkaline solutions could also be irritants. Edema may occur. Attempts to change flow rate such as applying pressure or a tourniquet have <u>no effect.</u> The catheter should be immediately removed, sterile dressings applied, and compresses used as well. The compresses should be warm for isotonic or normal pH solutions but cold if the solution is hypertonic or has an elevated pH.

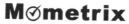

EXTRAVASATION

Extravasation is a complication that can occur when vesicant medications or solutions are infused. The term refers to the leaking of these solutions. Vesicants are substances capable of causing blistering if they leak into or are administered into tissue instead of the intended vessel. Subsequent shedding of tissue occurs. Complications can be severe including tissue death. Surgery is sometimes required if underlying tissues or bone structures become involved. A condition called reflex sympathetic dystrophy (RSD) where tissue is discolored can be found if permanent damage to tissues or nerves occurs. Symptoms are similar to those for infiltration, but in addition the solution flow rate usually decreases. If extravasation occurs, it is recommended to aspirate the remaining medication and blood and inject an antidote into the area before removing the catheter. The extremity should be elevated and cold compresses applied for alkylating or antibiotic vesicants, warm compresses applied for vinca alkaloids.

MECHANICAL COMPLICATIONS AFTER INSERTION WITH CENTRAL VASCULAR ACCESS DEVICES

After the insertion of a central vascular access device, the catheter or port can be dislodged after insertion and migrate to another area in the body. A common variant of this is called "Twiddler's syndrome" where the patient has the nervous habit of playing with the port and it becomes dislodged. Clinically symptoms can include swelling in the arm or shoulder or a burning sensation or pain upon infusion. In addition, the health care provider may observe things like an unusual length of the external catheter, coiling of the catheter under the skin, exposure of the cuff, leaking or difficulty with flow rate or aspiration. If the catheter is pulled out, then a sterile occlusive pressure dressing needs to be applied. If it is not, the position of the tip needs to be determined and repositioned. Any changes in intrathoracic pressure such as coughing, sneezing or forcing liquids through the catheter can also cause migration. This must be watched for possible congestive heart failure or thrombosis.

POOR PLACEMENT OF CENTRAL VASCULAR ACCESS DEVICE

When the catheter tip of a central vascular access device is **suboptimally placed**, a blood clot may form in a neck, chest or arm vessel. This often occurs with tunneled catheters on the left side. Thrombosis or blood clots occur because the flow of blood may stop, platelets can aggregate on the catheter surface resulting in injury to the vessel wall, or hypercoagulability often associated with malignancy may have occurred. The patient may experience pains in their chest, ear or jaw, swelling, lack of oxygen to the brain, emboli in the lungs, or bronchial obstruction. Since this catheter- related or vessel thrombosis as it referred to could lead to death, several precautions should be taken. Low-level anticoagulant therapy for patients at risk for clotting disorder should be administered. The right subclavian vein should be used if possible.

INCORRECT PLACEMENT OF CATHETER TIP INTRAVASCULARLY

Optimally, the catheter tip of a central vascular access device should be placed the vena cava. Sometimes due to anatomy the tip is **misplaced** into another intravascular space. This typically occurs when a tip intended to be inserted into the subclavian vein is misplaced into the internal jugular vein or the axillary vein is substituted for the cephalic vein. The patient often presents with discomfort or pain or edema in the neck, shoulder or arm regions, a gurgling sound running past the ear, or some type of neurological effect. Mechanically, the catheter is difficult to aspirate or infuse. Often these catheters can simply be repositioned especially if the patient can also be repositioned to accommodate this. Sometimes flushing with small amounts of saline can assist the repositioning. Direct fluoroscopic visualization by a radiologist is the best aid to use as an adjunct.

FORMATION OF FIBRIN ON CATHETER TIP

If **fibrin** forms on the catheter tip or along the access device where the catheter is in contact with the blood vessel, a clot develops and obstructs the catheter. A common cause is insufficient heparinization but others include some type of pump malfunction or break in the system, hypercoagulability, administration of medications that form precipitates, or some mechanical reason. The infusion will be sluggish or difficult and the blood foamy if aspirated. The patient may present with discomfort, pain or edema at or near the insertion site. Repositioning the patient and having them cough may help as well as flushing with saline. Other measures might include removing or cleaning a catheter with precipitate or use of a thrombolytic agent. If completely occluded, the health care provider cannot administer solutions or draw blood through these catheters.

OCCLUDED PERIPHERAL CATHETERS

When a catheter is jammed with blood or some type of precipitant, the solution flow is prevented or **occluded**. If the infusion rate decreases and it cannot be increased by mechanical measures, then occlusion has probably occurred. The occluded catheter should be removed and examined, dry and sterile dressings applied, and a new catheter placed in another vein. The potential for occlusion can be greatly diminished by a number of precautions including changing solutions when volume is less than 100 mL, checking medications and solutions for compatibility before mixing, flushing catheters with 0.9% saline, flushing with low concentrations of heparin in saline for central vascular access devices, and maintenance of positive pressure.

PHLEBITIS

Phlebitis is inflammation of a vein. If phlebitis is present, the insertion site and the vein are painful and tender or warm. There are three types of causes of phlebitis, chemical, mechanical, and bacterial:

- **Chemical causes** include administration of solutions with a high pH or a high solute concentration, or osmolality, of greater than 300 mOsm/L, rapid infusion rates, crystals resulting from improperly mixed medications, or presence of particles in the solution. This type of phlebitis can be diminished through use of filters, rotation of insertion sites, use of larger veins and smaller gauge needles in addition to proper delivery techniques.
- The material that the catheter is made of can sometimes cause the patient to develop **mechanical phlebitis**. This can also be caused by placement in flexion areas that causes irritation, use of large gauge needles, or poor securement of the device.
- A less common type of phlebitis, **bacterial phlebitis**, can occur with poor sterile technique, equipment, or insertion. However, this is can lead to septicemia. If this is suspected, catheters should be removed and cultured and another catheter placed in the opposite extremity.

POST-INFUSION PHLEBITIS

Post-infusion phlebitis refers to the vein inflammation or phlebitis that is not observable until after the catheter has been removed. Preventative measures coincide with those for any phlebitis. Since this complication could predispose the patient to infection including septicemia, a patient should always be monitored even after removing the catheter. Usually post-infusion phlebitis is observed within 48 hours if it occurs. At that time, cold or hot compresses should be applied, and medical interventions should be evaluated.

THROMBOSIS

Thrombosis occurs when an injury to the endothelial lining of the vein leads to the formation of a blood clot within that blood vessel. This occurs primarily because platelets will adhere to the battered wall forming a fibrinous clot. This blood clot formation can impair the circulation in the extremity where the insertion site is located so it is important to watch for the signs of thrombosis. The solution flow rate decreases because the space within the vein has narrowed and swelling of the extremity and surrounding area occurs. If thrombosis occurs or is suspected, the infusion should be discontinued immediately and the insertion site relocated to the opposite extremity if achievable. In order to decrease the flow of blood to the area, cold compresses should be temporarily applied.

PULMONARY EMBOLISM

When some type of mass of undissolved material floats and is deposited to the right side of the heart by the venous circulation, a pulmonary vessel can become occluded. This condition is a **pulmonary embolism**. The occluding material can be pieces of tissue, tumor cells, fats, air bubbles, bacteria or foreign material. A range of cardiac problems can result when the blockage obstructs the pulmonary artery. If the condition is suspected, the patient should be placed in the semi-Fowler's position and vital signs monitored. Treatments could include maintaining blood gas levels by administering oxygen and a heparin bolus followed by its infusion. A lung scan may be taken. Precautions like use of filters that retain either particulates or blood clots (for blood products), and not using veins in the lower extremities can reduce risk of pulmonary embolism.

AIR EMBOLISM

When a dose of air is introduced into the vascular system, bubbles that obstruct the pulmonary capillaries can result, called an **air embolism**, and generally acute distress is observed. This situation can occur if there is an open port or leak in the system, if the tubing is not clamped when the administration set is changed, if the Valsalva maneuver where the patient breathes out is not performed, or other measures to keep the solution running and free of air are not taken. Symptoms are generally rapid and acute and include chest pain, difficulty breathing, bluish skin, hypotension, increased pulse and ultimately shock with cardiac arrest if untreated. Obviously, the system should be replaced immediately, but in addition the patient should be placed on their left side with their head lower than the heart. Other measures such as monitoring vital signs and administering oxygen are usually done.

PIECE OF CATHETER ENTERING CIRCULATION

If a catheter is defective or somehow stripped during insertion, it can **break and enter the circulation** resulting in what is known as catheter embolism. Typically, this might be noticed if the catheter and hub separate or the severing is noticed upon withdrawal. Symptoms resemble those for other embolisms but can also include arrhythmias, perforation of the heart or endocarditis if the obstruction is stuck in the heart. Occasionally, there may be no apparent symptoms if the fragment lodges in the heart and other times the symptoms may be severe if a vein close to the heart such as the subclavian vein has been used. A tourniquet should be put on the arm above the insertion site and the patient confined to strict bed rest. The fragment needs to be identified by radiography and surgically removed.

PULMONARY EDEMA

When more fluid is introduced into the circulatory system than it can handle, the venous pressure is increased, the heart dilates, and a condition called **pulmonary edema** can result. If this occurs, initially the patient may have mild symptoms such as restlessness, shortness of breath, headache, cough or a mild increase in their pulse. As fluid builds up, though, they can develop hypertension, respirations may have a rippling sound, and the cough becomes productive. Eventually, they can develop symptoms like edema in the neck veins or eyelids, and ultimately heart failure, shock and cardiac arrest if left unrecognized. If a patient gains more than a pound a day, the health care provider should watch for other symptoms of pulmonary edema. Measures to relieve the heart's workload should be instituted when diagnosed, such as decreasing the infusion rate or giving the patient reagents like oxygen, morphine sulfate, diuretics or an IV vasodilator. Sometimes a therapeutic phlebotomy or incision is performed.

ALLERGIC REACTION TO MEDICATION OR SOLUTION

Before administration of solutions, medications, or blood products, history and blood tests documenting known allergies to medications, latex or iodine and blood group antigens should have already been done. If necessary, the patient should be wearing an allergy bracelet. If an **immediate or delayed allergic reaction** does occur, symptoms are typically chills and fever with or without a rash, redness, and itching of the skin. There could be shortness of breath and possible wheezing. After making the patient comfortable and notifying the physician, typical medications that might be ordered include antihistamines, epinephrine, cortisone or aminophylline. (Bronchodilator)

PNEUMOTHORAX

Pneumothorax is a complication that can arise when central venous catheters are used. The condition arises from puncturing of the pleural covering of the lung while putting the catheter in. Air enters the chest cavity and visceral pleura and air emboli can occur. The patient usually has a sudden onset of chest pain or shortness of breath and a crunching sound can be heard upon stethoscope examination. If severe, the patient has great difficulty breathing. The catheter should be removed immediately and the patient turned to the affected side and instructed to raise their arm. Oxygen is usually administered and a chest tube may be inserted.

COMPLICATIONS PRESENTING SIMILARLY TO PNEUMOTHORAX

Sudden onset of chest pain and shortness of breath upon insertion of a central venous catheter are hallmarks of pneumothorax, but these symptoms can also be associated with hemothorax or hydrothorax.

- **Hemothorax** is the term for the leakage of blood into the chest cavity as result of trauma or transection of a vein upon insertion.
- **Hydrothorax** is a situation that occurs when intravenous solutions are accidentally introduced right into the thoracic cavity, typically after transection of the subclavian vein. In this case vesicular breath sounds are absent and a flat-sounding murmur can be heard as well. This may require aspiration of the fluid from the pleural space.

A common reason for these situations is that the access device has been extravascularly malpositioned; in other words, the catheter has been placed or slipped outside the vein.

IDENTIFYING BRACHIAL PLEXUS INJURY OR ARTERIAL PUNCTURE

If a patient has a tingling sensation in their fingers or pain radiating down their arm, their **brachial plexus** might have been **punctured** during insertion. This complication could lead to paralysis in the extremity used. The brachial plexus is the network of nerves that supply the arm, forearm and hand. If bright red blood is withdrawn from the insertion needle, an artery may have been inadvertently punctured. This could lead to a hematoma, compression of the trachea, respiratory distress, or a central nervous system effects if a blot clot or other emboli in the brain has occurred. In most cases, pressure needs to be applied to the site for at least 5 minutes.

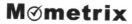

PERICARDIAL TAMPONADE

If a centrally placed catheter pierces the atrium, excess fluid will accumulate in the pericardium, which is the membrane that surrounds the heart, causing what is called **pericardial tamponade**. Symptoms are delayed until enough blood or solution leaks into the space to compress the heart, resulting in a condition called pericardial tamponade. The cardiovascular system shuts down as signaled by possible neck vein distention, a narrow pulse pressure, and hypotension. Other symptoms of heart failure may be absent. Emergency intervention is crucial including aspiration of the pericardial sac just below the sternum's xiphoid process and resuscitation.

SUPERIOR VENA CAVA SYNDROME

If the superior vena cava (SVC) is occluded or compressed, the flow of blood becomes impossible and a condition called **superior vena cava syndrome** results. This condition is usually caused by a blood clot, fibrin formation or the combination of the two developing an occlusion. Sometimes, however, the same syndrome results when a tumor or an enlarged lymph node presses against the SVC. The patient develops a progressive shortness of breath or cough, edema in the upper body, cyanosis in the face or other upper regions, engorged and distended veins, headache and visual or mental changes. Loss of blood to the brain and bronchial obstruction can develop and if left untreated ultimately death is possible. Oxygen should be administered to the patient and anticoagulant therapy is generally begun.

ARTERIAL OR VENOUS SPASMS

When a patient experiences numbness in the extremity where a catheter has been inserted or cramping and pain above the insertion site, they may have had an **arterial or venous spasm**. The usual causative agents are use of cold or irritating medications or solutions or an accidental puncture of the blood vessel. These spasms are involuntary contractions of the artery or vein that temporarily stop the blood flow in that vessel. Arterial spasms are the most serious because the arteries deliver blood to large areas of the body, pulse may be lost, and therefore tissue necrosis and gangrene could occur if unattended. The catheter should be immediately removed and pressure applied to the site for about 5 minutes. If a venous spasm occurs, less blood supply is cut off, so the catheter is usually not removed. Instead measures like decreasing the rate, diluting the medication, applying warm compresses, or assuaging the pain with lidocaine are more common.

COMPLICATIONS TO IMPLANTED DEVICES IN PATIENTS WITH WEIGHT LOSS OR POOR NUTRITION

In patients who are extremely thin, have a poor nutritional status or experience significant weight loss, the skin over the portal septum of their implanted catheter or other device may tear. A condition called **skin erosion**, which is basically visible rubbing or tears possibly accompanied by redness or swelling, results. This can also happen if some type of trauma occurs, such as the patient falling or being injured. The device is usually removed if this occurs, and the skin area treated to prevent infection and covered with a sterile dressing.

CRNI Practice Test

1. According to the Institute of Medicine's definition of evidence-based practice, the most relevant research is

    a. epidemiological.
    b. patient-centered clinical.
    c. qualitative data collection.
    d. basic medical/experimental.

2. In evidence-based practice, the best description of patient preference is

    a. an essential component.
    b. a secondary component.
    c. an intervening component.
    d. an optional component.

3. Which of the following is the most critical element in preventing infections associated with venous access devices?

    a. Hand hygiene
    b. Device selection
    c. Insertion site protection
    d. Health professional's experience

4. Which of the following intravenous drugs is incompatible with intravenous morphine sulfate?

    a. Fentanyl citrate
    b. Famotidine
    c. Furosemide
    d. Fluconazole

5. Which is the preferred method to prevent movement and catheter migration associated with a venous access device?

    a. Suturing in place
    b. Securing with transparent dressing
    c. Securing with sterile tape
    d. Securing with a catheter stabilization device

6. A patient is admitted to the unit after vomiting excessively for 4 days at home. The patient's serum pH is elevated, PCO_2 is relatively normal, and urine pH is >6. The patient is dizzy, confused and is exhibiting tremors, seizures, tingling, tachycardia, arrhythmias, and hypoventilation. The patient is most likely exhibiting symptoms of

    a. respiratory alkalosis.
    b. metabolic alkalosis.
    c. respiratory acidosis.
    d. metabolic acidosis.

7. Which of the following veins should be avoided for short peripheral catheter insertion?

a. Metacarpal vein
b. Cephalic vein
c. Antecubital fossa vein
d. Basilic vein

8. Which of the following does the Occupational Safety and Health Administration (OSHA) regulate?

a. Patient right to privacy
b. Disposal methods for sharps, such as needles
c. Reimbursement for services
d. Patient surveys

9. According to the phlebitis scale, when a streak and/or palpable venous cord begins to form, the phlebitis is classified as which of the following?

a. Grade 1
b. Grade 2
c. Grade 3
d. Grade 4

10. Which of the following is a normal serum osmolality for an adult patient?

a. 285 mOsm/kg
b. 270mOsm/kg
c. 310 mOsm/kg
d. 265 mOsm/kg

11. A palliative care patient requires intravenous therapy for about 6 to 8 weeks. Which of the following central venous access devices is most commonly used for this duration?

a. Non-tunneled central catheter
b. Peripherally-inserted central catheter (PICC)
c. Tunneled central catheter
d. Implantable port

12. The infusion nurse is teaching a patient to manage his pain pump for patient-controlled analgesia (PCA). Although the nurse explains at least 3 times, the patient asks the same questions over and over. The nurse provides a pamphlet with illustrations, but the patient barely looks at them and states he can't figure out what he needs to do. The next best approach is probably to

a. suggest a different method of pain control.
b. arrange for someone else to manage the equipment.
c. allow a rest period and then start again with instructions.
d. allow the patient to practice with actual equipment.

13. Parenteral nutrition with a total nutrient admixture that includes lipids has been ordered for a burn patient for administration over a 24-hour period. When preparing to administer the solution, the infusion nurse observes that the oil has separated, forming an obvious layer. Which is the correct action?

   a. Administer the solution, as oil separation is normal
   b. Mix the solution by shaking the bag until no oil separation is noticeable
   c. Discard the solution
   d. Return the solution to the pharmacy for addition of added emulsifier

14. A 4-year-old child has had severe diarrhea and vomiting for 3 days. Which of the following indicates isotonic dehydration?

   a. Sunken eyeballs, subnormal temperature, lethargy, skin dry and turgor poor, and tachycardia
   b. Severe thirst, skin turgor fair, tremors, hyperirritability, and muscle rigidity
   c. Seizures, coma, cold clammy skin, poor skin turgor, and tachycardic, thready pulse
   d. Peripheral edema, apathy, hypertension, and moist cough

15. During intermittent administration of antibiotics through a secondary intravenous (piggyback) set (gravity infusion), the secondary set should be positioned

   a. at the same level as the primary set.
   b. above the primary set.
   c. below the primary set.
   d. in any position.

16. Only an adult medication is available for pediatric dosing for a 3-year-old child. If the pediatric dose volume is 0.08 mL, which of the following actions is indicated?

   a. Prepare a 1:10 dilution
   b. Prepare a 1:150 dilution
   c. Prepare a 1:100 dilution
   d. Do not administer drug

17. When positioning a toddler (1 to 3) for a procedure, which of the following positions is most likely to cause the child fear?

   a. Fetal
   b. Side-lying
   c. Prone
   d. Supine

18. A patient who receives multiple transfusions with citrated blood products must be monitored closely for

   a. hyponatremia.
   b. hypomagnesemia.
   c. hypokalemia.
   d. hypocalcemia.

19. In a patient receiving total parenteral nutrition, which of the following is an indication of essential fatty acid deficiency?
    a. Thrombocytosis
    b. Pernicious anemia
    c. Hemolytic anemia
    d. Iron deficiency anemia

20. When a gauze dressing is applied to contain bleeding about a catheter exit site under a transparent dressing, how frequently should the complete dressing be changed?
    a. Every 24 hours
    b. Every 48 hours
    c. Every 72 hours
    d. Every 7 days

21. Which is the correct position to place a patient who will have a central venous catheter inserted through a subclavian approach?
    a. Fowler's
    b. Reverse Trendelenburg
    c. Trendelenburg
    d. Semi-Fowler's

22. A patient develops sudden fever and chills, nausea, diarrhea, vomiting, hypotension, and tachycardia within 6 hours of receiving parenteral fluids. Which of the following is recommended to rule out septicemia related to the central catheter?
    a. Culture of parenteral fluids
    b. Cultures of peripheral blood and blood per catheter
    c. Culture of blood per catheter
    d. Culture of IV administration set and fluid container

23. Chemotherapeutic drugs that are classified as vesicants, which can cause severe tissue damage, include
    a. mitomycin, dactinomycin, and vinblastine.
    b. bleomycin, carboplatin, and fluorouracil.
    c. dacarbazine and streptozocin.
    d. cyclophosphamide, cytarabine, and asparaginase.

24. During administration of the chemotherapeutic agent vinblastine, extravasation occurs. Which of the following antidotes is indicated?
    a. 10% sodium thiosulfate
    b. Dimethyl sulfoxide (DMSO)
    c. Totect® (dexrazoxane)
    d. Recombinant hyaluronidase (Hylenex®)

25. When administering intravenous push medications through a patient's infusion set, the purpose of occluding the intravenous line by pinching the tubing above the injection port is to

    a. flush the tubing.
    b. aspirate for return of blood.
    c. ensure medication is given as a bolus.
    d. check for occlusion.

26. Packed red blood cells can be refrigerated for

    a. no more than 5 days.
    b. no more than 42 days.
    c. 10 years.
    d. 1 year.

27. The nurse must insert a peripheral line, but the patient's arms and hands are excessively hairy. Which is the best solution?

    a. Remove the excess hair with scissors or surgical clippers
    b. Wash the skin with soap and water before using antiseptic
    c. Use a depilatory agent
    d. Shave with a razor

28. Normovolemic hemodilution for surgery involves which of the following?

    a. Administering extra intravenous fluid to dilute the blood to decrease loss of blood cells with bleeding
    b. Administering intravenous fluid in the approximate amount of blood loss during surgery
    c. Withdrawing blood prior to surgery, replacing it with intravenous fluid, and then reinfusing the blood after surgery
    d. Withdrawing blood prior to surgery and then reinfusing it along with replacement intravenous fluid after surgery

29. When teaching a chemotherapy patient at risk for neutropenia, which dietary restriction should be advised?

    a. Fresh fruits
    b. Dairy products
    c. High fiber vegetables
    d. Meats

30. A patient receiving platelet transfusions develops sudden onset of chills, fever, headache, flushing, anxiety and muscle aches but does not have respiratory distress, and blood pressure is within normal range. The most likely cause is

    a. acute hemolytic reaction.
    b. mild allergic reaction.
    c. severe allergic reaction.
    d. febrile nonhemolytic reaction.

31. When preparing a unit of packed red blood cells for administration, the nurse notes that gas bubbles are present in the unit. Which of the following is correct?
   a. The PRBCs may be contaminated with bacteria
   b. The PRBCs may be undergoing hemolysis
   c. The PRBCs are normal
   d. The PRBCs may contain excess plasma

32. When inserting a midline catheter in the arm, the nurse encounters resistance while advancing the catheter and stops. Which next action is correct?
   a. Immediately remove catheter
   b. Continue to slowly advance catheter while flushing with NS
   c. Change angle of arm or wrist and/or ask the patient to make and release a fist
   d. Flush catheter with NS

33. According to the infiltration scale, if the skin is blanched and cool and edema extends less than one inch from the insertion point, what grade is the infiltration?
   a. Grade 1
   b. Grade 2
   c. Grade 3
   d. Grade 4

34. In order to increase plasma volume by one liter, which of the following requires the smallest volume of fluid replacement?
   a. 0.9% NS
   b. 3% NS
   c. 5% colloid
   d. 25% colloid

35. A patient who has been receiving intravenous furosemide complains of anorexia, nausea, and muscle weakness. Examination shows hypotension, and on interview the patient appears lethargic and is slightly confused. Which of the following electrolyte imbalances is most likely?
   a. Hyponatremia
   b. Hypocalcemia
   c. Hypokalemia
   d. Hypomagnesemia

36. Which of the following positive signs can indicate the presence of tetany related to hypocalcemia and hypomagnesemia?
   a. Trousseau's sign
   b. Kernig's sign
   c. Romberg's sign
   d. Psoas sign

37. Which of the following allergies places a patient at risk for anaphylactic reaction to IV protamine?

    a. Milk products
    b. Tree nuts
    c. Soy
    d. Fish products

38. Flumazenil should be available as a reversal agent for which of the following drugs commonly used for conscious sedation?

    a. Fentanyl
    b. Droperidol
    c. Midazolam
    d. Propofol

39. What is the minimal urinary output per hour expected for an adult patient?

    a. 20 mL
    b. 30 mL
    c. 40 mL
    d. 50 mL

40. Which of the following medications may be used as pretreatment prior to administration of chemotherapeutic agents to reduce incidence of nausea and vomiting?

    a. Famotidine
    b. Prochlorperazine
    c. Lorazepam
    d. Metoclopramide

41. A patient's lab reports shows a slightly elevated total white blood count with equal elevations of all types of white blood cells, an elevated hemoglobin and hematocrit, normal creatinine but elevated blood-urea-nitrogen, increased urine specific gravity, and increased serum sodium. The most likely nursing diagnosis is

    a. risk for infection.
    b. deficient fluid volume.
    c. excess fluid volume.
    d. imbalanced nutrition.

42. Adult central venous catheters should be flushed with

    a. 10 mL 0.9% sodium chloride or 5% glucose.
    b. 5 mL 0.9% sodium chloride or 5% glucose.
    c. heparin 10 units/mL.
    d. heparin 100 units/mL.

43. Which type of infusion pump is most appropriate for large-volume infusion of crystalloids?

    a. Syringe pump
    b. APO-go pump
    c. Volumetric pump
    d. Multi-channel pump

44. The care bundle to prevent infection from central lines includes which of the following?

    a. Laboratory monitoring
    b. Weekly review of necessity of all lines
    c. Alcohol skin cleansing
    d. Hand hygiene and barrier precautions

45. Which of the following is an example of intrinsic contamination of intravenous fluids?

    a. Contamination occurs during admixture procedures
    b. Contamination occurs during manufacturing
    c. Contamination occurs because of inadequate storage and refrigeration
    d. Contamination occurs because of improper technique

46. Excessive hypotonic intravenous fluids may result in which of the following fluid imbalances?

    a. Extracellular fluid volume deficit (ECFVD)
    b. Extracellular fluid volume shift (ECFV Shift)
    c. Intracellular fluid volume excess (ICFVE)
    d. Extracellular fluid volume excess (ECFVE)

47. If using an intravenous set with a Standard Drop Factor of 15 drops per mL, what is the flow rate in drops per minute needed to administer 1 liter of fluid over a 5-hour period?

    a. 180 drops/min
    b. 90 drops/min
    c. 60 drops/min
    d. 50 drops/min

48. The flow rate of an intravenous solution administered per gravity is directly proportional to

    a. the length of tubing.
    b. the viscosity of IV fluid.
    c. the height of the liquid column (fluid container).
    d. the temperature of the infusion.

49. For a severely burned adult patient receiving total parenteral nutrition (TPN), nitrogen supplementation may be up to

    a. 0.8 g/kg per day.
    b. 1 g/kg per day.
    c. 1.5 g/kg per day.
    d. 2.5 g/kg per day.

50. A patient receiving paclitaxel develops a hypersensitivity reaction (non-anaphylactic) during administration. Which of the following initial actions is correct?

    a. Stop infusion and discontinue IV
    b. Stop infusion and administer corticosteroid
    c. Stop infusion and administer epinephrine
    d. Stop infusion and provide rapid infusion of NS

51. Power injectable catheters are specifically designed to accommodate

a. RBCs.
b. WBCs.
c. contrast medium (CT).
d. chemotherapeutic agents.

52. How long can a midline peripheral catheter stay in place?

a. 1 to 2 weeks
b. 2 to 4 weeks
c. 4 to 6 weeks
d. 6 to 8 weeks

53. Which of the following drugs or fluids can safely be administered through a short peripheral catheter?

a. Vinblastine
b. 20% dextrose in water (D20W)
c. 5% dextrose in water (D5W)
d. Doxorubicin

54. Under the CDC's standard precautions, hand hygiene must be carried out

a. before every patient contact.
b. before and after every patient contact.
c. before and after contact with infected patients.
d. before patient contact that involves patient touching only.

55. Which of the following is an indication for a CVAD?

a. Chemotherapy scheduled for greater than 3 months
b. Patient's clinical condition is stabilizing
c. Infusions required for greater than one week
d. Patient requires transfusions for blood loss from fractured pelvis

56. If a patient has small veins and the CRNI is unable to access a peripheral vein in the hand or forearm, what is the best solution?

a. Access a vein the foot
b. Access a vein in the antecubital area
c. Recommend a CVAD
d. Use ultrasound to assist in accessing the vein

57. If using ultrasound guidance to locate a vein for cannulation, how can the CRNI differentiate an artery from a vein?

a. The artery compresses more easily than the vein
b. The vein pulsates under pressure
c. The vein compresses but the artery does not
d. The artery is larger than the vein

58. If a patient is hypovolemic and anticipated IV replacement fluid volume is 2 to 3 L, which IV fluid is usually the first choice?

a. NS
b. D5W
c. Lactated Ringers
d. D5 ½ NS

59. Which of the following IV fluids is usually used for a patient that is NPO and receiving maintenance fluids pre-procedure?

a. NS
b. D5 ½ NS
c. ½ NS
d. Plasmalyte

60. What does a *soft limit* on a smart pump refer to?

a. An alert that the CRNI cannot override
b. An alert that the CRNI can override
c. A volume that can be adjusted
d. A preset volume that cannot be adjusted

61. Which of the following IV fluids is most appropriate for fluid replacement in a patient with extensive 2nd and 3rd degree burns?

a. D5W
b. 10DW
c. NS
d. Lactated Ringers

62. When selecting a catheter for a PICC line, what is the most appropriate catheter-to-vein ratio?

a. ≤35%
b. ≤45%
c. ≤55%
d. ≤65%

63. The three factors in Virchow's triad that relate to catheter-associated thrombus formation are

a. vascular injury, altered blood flow, and hypercoagulability.
b. vascular inflammation, altered blood flow, and hypocoagulability.
c. vascular injury, hypovolemia, and infection.
d. vascular inflammation, hypovolemia, and hypercoagulability.

64. If a patient with pancreatic cancer will require long-term intermittent antineoplastic chemotherapy, which of the following is the recommended access device?

a. Midline catheter
b. Cuffed, tunneled CVAD
c. Implanted vascular access port
d. PICC.

65. Which of the following is a contraindication for insertion of a PICC line?
  a. Chronic liver disease
  b. Chronic heart disease
  c. Malignancy
  d. Chronic kidney disease

66. If taking a blood sample from a PICC line after flushing, how much blood should be discarded before taking the sample?
  a. None
  b. 2 mL
  c. 5 mL
  d. 10 mL

67. When therapeutic phlebotomy is utilized to treat conditions such as polycythemia vera, hemochromatosis, or porphyria, about what volume of blood is usually withdrawn with each treatment?
  a. 100 mL
  b. 250 mL
  c. 300 mL
  d. 450 mL

68. In the chain of infection, how can healthcare providers break the portal of entry link?
  a. Pasteurization and disinfection
  b. Quarantine or medical treatment
  c. Face mask and gloves
  d. Vaccinations and improved nutrition.

69. What is a primary difference between veins and arteries?
  a. The walls of veins have 3 layers
  b. The lumens of veins have a lesser diameter
  c. Arteries can serve as blood reservoirs
  d. The middle layer of the vein wall is poorly developed

70. A patient suffering from oxygen deprivation develops cyanosis because of
  a. high concentration of deoxyhemoglobin in the blood.
  b. low concentration of deoxyhemoglobin in the blood.
  c. high concentration of oxyhemoglobin in the blood.
  d. increased death rate of red blood cells.

71. The normal pH of the blood ranges from
  a. 5.35 to 5.45.
  b. 6.35 to 6.45.
  c. 7.35 to 7.45.
  d. 8.35 to 7.45.

72. **Extracellular fluids constitute what percentage volume of total body water?**
    a. 25%
    b. 37%
    c. 75%
    d. 63%

73. **In which part of the brain is the thirst center located that regulates the sensation of thirst to maintain water balance in the body?**
    a. Cerebral cortex
    b. Pituitary gland
    c. Brainstem
    d. Hypothalamus

74. **How long after a patient receives a hazardous drug, such as an antineoplastic agent, should the CRNI use extra precautions when handling or exposed to the patient's bodily fluids?**
    a. 6 hours
    b. 12 hours
    c. 24 hours
    d. 48 hours

75. **If a patient has a large wound infected with MRSA, what type of precautions is indicated?**
    a. Standard only
    b. Contact
    c. Droplet
    d. Airborne

76. **The preferred vein for venipuncture to obtain a blood sample with the H-shaped vein distribution pattern is generally the**
    a. median cubital vein.
    b. cephalic vein.
    c. basilic vein.
    d. intermediate antebrachial vein.

77. **Venipuncture of the basilic vein is usually avoided because**
    a. the vein is too small.
    b. of risk of accidental puncture of a nerve.
    c. the vein cannot be visualized.
    d. the vein is difficult to palpate.

78. **According to the order of the draw established by the CLSI, which of the following blood samples would be obtained first?**
    a. Heparin tube with gel plasma separator
    b. EDTA tube
    c. Sterile tube (blood culture)
    d. Blue-top coagulation tube

79. If preparing an IV infusion of a chemotherapeutic agent that has splash potential, which PPE is required?

   a. Double gloves, gown, and eye protection
   b. Gloves and gown
   c. Double gloves, gown, eye protection, and respiratory protection
   d. Double gloves and eye protection

80. If, when preparing a chemotherapeutic agent for IV infusion, the CRNI accidentally spills approximately 10 mL of the drug in the safety cabinet, what is the first step?

   a. Utilize the spill kit
   b. Notify the safety director
   c. Clear all people from the area
   d. Sound the emergency alarm

81. How many mL of blood are generally needed for ABG analysis?

   a. 0.5 mL
   b. 1 mL
   c. 1.5 mL
   d. 2 mL

82. Which of the following electrolytes is likely to increase after multiple blood transfusions?

   a. Carbon dioxide
   b. Chloride
   c. Sodium
   d. Potassium

83. Which type of hypersensitivity reaction is associated with blood transfusion incompatibility reactions?

   a. Type I
   b. Type II
   c. Type III
   d. Type IV

84. The IV administration of an immediate-use compounded sterile product (CSP) must be initiated within

   a. 15 minutes.
   b. 30 minutes.
   c. 60 minutes.
   d. 90 minutes.

85. Which of the following is associated with shorter catheter survival time for short peripheral catheters?

   a. Long 12 cm catheter length
   b. Vein depth of 1 cm
   c. Vein diameter
   d. Short 5 cm catheter length

86. Near-infrared (nIR) light devices are appropriate to aid in

    a. cannulation of superficial peripheral veins.
    b. cannulation of internal jugular vein.
    c. arterial puncture in adults.
    d. insertion of femoral CVADs.

87. What type of needle must be used to access an implanted CVA port?

    a. Standard point
    b. Venting
    c. Hypodermic
    d. Huber point

88. If using the Vein Entry Indicator Device® (VEID), how does the device indicate penetration of a vein?

    a. Vein illuminates
    b. Device beeps
    c. Device flashes a light
    d. Device buzzes

89. For a CVAD with an upper body insertion site, the tip should be located

    a. near the superior cavoatrial junction.
    b. near the tricuspid valve.
    c. in the right ventricle.
    d. in the inferior vena cava.

90. In order to utilize ECG tip confirmation for insertion of a CVAD, which of the following must be present?

    a. P waves
    b. T waves
    c. Normal sinus rhythm
    d. Pulse rate <100 bpm

91. If vesicant (anthracycline) extravasation occurs, the CRNI should immediately

    a. stop the infusion and remove the needle.
    b. stop the infusion and aspirate the vesicant.
    c. stop the infusion and apply a warm compress.
    d. Stop the infusion and apply cold compresses.

92. A blood warmer can be used with which of the following blood components?

    a. Red blood cells and platelets
    b. Red blood cells and cryoprecipitate
    c. Red blood cells and granulocytes
    d. Red blood cells

93. When a patient is undergoing plasmapheresis/therapeutic plasma exchange, for which of the following complications should the CRNI be especially on alert?

    a. Infection
    b. Electrolyte imbalance
    c. Hypovolemia
    d. Hypervolemia

94. When administering platelets to a patient, the infusion should be done

    a. as quickly as possible.
    b. as slowly as possible.
    c. over 1-2 hours.
    d. over 2-4 hours.

95. The basic maintenance fluid requirement for parenteral formulations for the first 20 kg of weight for adults is

    a. 20-25 mL/kg/d.
    b. 25-30 mL/kg/d.
    c. 30-35 mL/kg/d.
    d. 35-40 mL/kg/d.

96. When using a primary infusion set with a secondary (piggyback) set, what is the purpose of the check valve?

    a. Control the size of the droplet
    b. Control the drop factor
    c. Remove foreign particles
    d. Prevent retrograde flow of solution

97. A secondary (piggyback) administration set can deliver up to

    a. 100 mL.
    b. 250 mL.
    c. 500 mL.
    d. 1000 mL.

98. What is a risk especially associated with the use of a primary Y administration set?

    a. Hemolysis
    b. Air embolism
    c. Obstruction
    d. Contamination

99. If a patient with hyperemesis gravidarum has an order for IV dextrose solution because of hypoglycemia and dehydration, the CRNI should verify that the patient has received

    a. thiamine.
    b. antiemetic.
    c. vitamin D.
    d. cobalamin.

100. With a needleless connector with positive fluid displacement, it is important to
   a. clamp the catheter before or after disconnection.
   b. clamp the catheter before disconnection.
   c. clamp the catheter after disconnection.
   d. avoid clamping the catheter.

101. What type of filter would be appropriate for reinfusion of autologous blood retrieved during surgery involving extensive blood loss?
   a. Leukocyte reduction filter
   b. Microaggregate filter
   c. Standard clot filter, 170 microns
   d. Standard clot filter, 260 microns

102. The most common type of CVAD is the
   a. non-tunneled CVAD.
   b. tunneled CVAD.
   c. implanted port.
   d. PICC.

103. When receiving IV fluids, older adults are most at risk for
   a. hypervolemic hyponatremia.
   b. hypervolemic hypernatremia.
   c. hypovolemic hypernatremia.
   d. hypovolemic hyponatremia.

104. Femoral catheters for vascular access for hemodialysis for patients with chronic renal failure should be left in place for no longer than
   a. 2 days.
   b. 5 days.
   c. 2 weeks.
   d. 4 weeks.

105. In order to reduce the risk of CLABSI from non-tunneled CVADs in adults, which vein is preferred?
   a. Jugular
   b. Femoral
   c. Cephalic
   d. Subclavian

106. If using a use-activated container to administer an IV drug, it is essential that the CRNI
   a. ensure complete rupture of the reservoir.
   b. avoid applying pressure to the container.
   c. rotate the container to mix the solutions.
   d. use a vented administration set.

107. The occlusion alarm on an EID indicates

a. air in the line.
b. dry container.
c. fluid not flowing.
d. low battery.

108. When preparing a patient for insertion of a tunneled catheter into the internal jugular vein, what position should the patient be placed in?

a. Flat, supine
b. 10-15° Trendelenburg
c. Low Fowler's position
d. High Fowler's position

109. If a patient is receiving total parenteral nutrition (TPN), fat emulsions should generally not exceed a maximum dose of

a. 1 g/kg/d.
b. 1.5 g/kg/d.
c. 2 g/kg/d.
d. 2.5 g/kg/d.

110. If a patient is receiving total parenteral nutrition (TPN) and develops dermatitis, hair loss, anorexia, immunocompromise, stomatitis, glossitis, and depressed healing, what trace mineral deficiency does this indicate?

a. Zinc
b. Manganese
c. Selenium
d. Copper

111. If the CRNI is unable to insert an IV to provide fluids into a child dehydrated from diarrhea, the best alternative is likely

a. CVAD.
b. hypodermoclysis.
c. oral fluids.
d. rectal instillation.

112. If administering infusate in a glass container, which type of administration set is required?

a. Filtered
b. Gravity
c. Non-vented
d. Vented

113. With CRBSI, the source of the infection is

a. intrinsic factors.
b. extrinsic factors.
c. the catheter itself.
d. any factor.

124

Copyright © Mometrix Media. You have been licensed one copy of this document for personal use only. Any other reproduction or redistribution is strictly prohibited. All rights reserved.

114. When a child is utilizing patient-controlled analgesia (PCA), the limit (total dosage that can be delivered in a set duration of time) is usually set at

   a.   12 hours.
   b.   8 hours.
   c.   6 hours.
   d.   4 hours.

115. The primary use for peristaltic pumps is for

   a.   enteral feedings.
   b.   blood components.
   c.   contrast medium.
   d.   maintenance fluids.

116. Which of the following should be avoided with plastic administration sets that include DEHP (a plasticizer that makes the sets pliable)?

   a.   Platelets
   b.   Lipid-based solutions
   c.   Dextrose containing solutions
   d.   Antibiotics

117. Which of the following is the preferred vascular access device for patients with chronic kidney disease requiring hemodialysis?

   a.   AV fistula
   b.   AV graft
   c.   long-term VAD
   d.   Implantable port

118. If using a transillumination device, such as the Venoscope®, what is the first thing the CRNI should do when a dark line appears between the arms of the device?

   a.   Outline the vein with a surgical marking pen
   b.   Secure the device in place with Velcro bands
   c.   Apply pressure to both arms of the device and observe the dark line
   d.   Hold the device in place and insert the needle

119. Which of the following is associated with increased risk of infection with total parenteral nutrition (TPN)?

   a.   Overfeeding
   b.   Underfeeding
   c.   Hypoglycemia
   d.   Hypervolemia

120. An EID is unable to detect

   a.   malfunctioning.
   b.   incorrectly loaded tubing.
   c.   dry container.
   d.   infiltration.

Answer Key and Explanations

1. B: Patient-centered clinical research is the most relevant research for the development of evidence-based practice. The clinical research can be interventional or observational but centers on the needs and responses of the patient. **Epidemiological research** focuses on historical patterns in the frequency and distribution of disease. **Qualitative data collection**, often used in the beginning phases of research exploration, utilizes focus groups, interviews, and narrative reports to gain information. **Basic medical/Experimental research** focuses on health-related topics, such as biochemistry and genetics, and may include animal experimentation.

2. A: Patient preference is an essential component of EBP because the values and preferences of the patient affect the patient's willingness to cooperate and participate as well as the patient's recovery. Patient preferences should always be considered as part of the plan of care and the plan developed in partnership with the patient. When patients choose a treatment option or plan of care not supported by evidence, then the nurse must provide unbiased information. Other essential components of EBP include best practices (based on clinical research), clinical experience/expertise, and context (including the setting and patient situation).

3. A: Hand hygiene is the most critical element in preventing infection associated with venous access devices. Hands that are dirty or contaminated with body fluids (feces, urine, blood) should be washed thoroughly (minimum 15 seconds) with antimicrobial or non-antimicrobial soap and water. If hands are not visibly dirty, then an alcohol hand rub may be used, following manufacturer's recommendations. Hands should be decontaminated prior to and after any direct contact with a patient and before application and after removal of sterile gloves.

4. C: Furosemide is incompatible with morphine sulfate. Incompatibility occurs if when two drugs are mixed together, chemical deterioration occurs in of one or both drugs. Incompatibility may be physical or chemical. In some cases, precipitates may form or the solution may appear hazy or discolored, but these obvious changes are not always present, so drug compatibility must always be verified. Effects may be synergistic or antagonistic, or some new effect may occur.

5. D: A catheter stabilization device is the preferred method to prevent movement and catheter migration associated with venous access devices. Stabilizing reduces the risk of phlebitis and infection. Suturing is associated with higher infection rates as it is more invasive. Sterile tapes can provide adequate stabilization but may loosen if the patient is diaphoretic or bleeding occurs at insertion site. The stabilization device should be changed with routine catheter care.

6. B: These symptoms are typical of metabolic alkalosis: Elevated serum pH, PCO_2 relatively normal (if compensated) or increased (if uncompensated), and urine pH >6 (if compensated). The patient is dizzy, confused and is exhibiting tremors, seizures, tingling, tachycardia, arrhythmias. Metabolic alkalosis occurs with decreased strong acid or increased base, with compensatory CO_2 retention by the lungs associated with hypoventilation. Metabolic alkalosis is usually caused by excessive vomiting, gastric suctioning, diuretics, potassium deficit, excessive mineralocorticoids, and/or excessive $NaHCO_3$ intake.

7. C: The antecubital fossa veins should be avoided for short peripheral catheter insertion because they are in an area of flexion, which can result in phlebitis or infiltration. Also, because antecubital fossa veins are easily accessible, they should be saved and other veins used first. The most distal veins should be used first although insertion should be proximal to previous insertion sites. Veins often used for short peripheral catheters include metacarpal, median, cephalic, and basilic veins.

8. B: The Occupational Safety and Health Administration (OSHA) regulates workplace safety, including disposal methods for sharps, such as needles. OSHA requires that standard precautions be used at all times and that staff be trained to use precautions. OSHA requires procedures for post-exposure evaluation and treatment and availability of hepatitis B vaccine for healthcare workers. OSHA defines occupational exposure to infections, establishes standards to prevent the spread of bloodborne pathogens, and regulates the fitting and use of respirators.

9. C: Grade 3. Phlebitis may occur because of irritating medications or IV fluids, injury to the lining of the vein, or infection. The phlebitis scale:

- Grade 0: Asymptomatic.
- Grade 1: Redness about site and may complain of pain.
- Grade 2: Pain as well as redness and/or swelling.
- Grade 3: Pain and redness as well as streak and/or palpable venous cord.
- Grade 4: Pain and redness as well as streak and palpable venous cord more than one inch long and/or purulent discharge.

10. A: A normal serum osmolality for an adult patient is 285 mOsm/kg (normal range 275 to 300 mOsm/kg). Hypo-osmolality occurs with values <275 mOsm/kg (critical value 265 mOsm/g) and hyper-osmolality with values above 300 mOsm/kg (critical value 320 mOsm/kg). When sodium levels increase or fluid levels decrease, osmolality increases. Corticosteroid and mannitol may increase serum osmolality while carbamazepine, hydrochlorothiazide, and chlorpromazine may decrease levels. Respiratory arrest may result from levels of 360 mOsm/kg. Death may occur with levels >420 mOsm/g.

11. B: Peripherally-inserted central catheters (PICCs) are frequently used for intravenous infusions over several days or months (intermediate-term). PICC lines are used for chemotherapy and are inserted in one of the arms, usually below the elbow. **Non-tunneled central catheters** are used for short-term therapy, usually under 6 weeks. **Tunneled central catheters** are inserted when patients require long-term intravenous therapy as they may stay in place for many years. **Implantable ports** are also used primarily for long-term IV therapy. Once implanted, the ports require little care and are easily accessed.

12. D: The patient's inability to understand oral instructions and disinterest in illustrations suggests a **kinesthetic learner**, so the nurse should allow the patient to handle the equipment and practice. Kinesthetic learns learn best by handling, doing, and practicing with minimal directions and hands-on experience. Other learning styles include:

Visual learner learns best by seeing and reading:

- Provide written directions, picture guides, or demonstrate procedures.
- Use charts and diagrams.
- Provide photos, videos.

Auditory learner learns best by listening and talking:

- Explain procedures while demonstrating and have learner repeat.
- Plan extra time to discuss and answer questions.
- Provide audiotapes.

13. C: The total nutrient admixture should be discarded if there is "cracking" of the lipid emulsion and the oil separates into a layer. With TPN, all the components of parenteral nutrition and lipids are admixed together in one container to create a 3-in-1 formula. Components of parenteral nutrition generally include proteins, carbohydrates, fats, electrolytes, vitamins, sterile water, and trace vitamins. While most postoperative patients need 1500 calories per day to prevent protein breakdown, those with fever, burns, major surgery, trauma, or hypermetabolic disease may need up to 10,000 more calories daily.

14. A: Isotonic dehydration is the most common type occurring in children (up to 70%) with severe diarrhea. Indications include sunken eyeballs, subnormal temperature (except with an active infection), lethargy, skin dry and turgor poor, thirst, marked weight loss, and tachycardia. Sodium levels are within normal range. Longitudinal furrows may be noted on the tongue. Infants may exhibit depressed fontanels. In isotonic dehydration, water and electrolytes are lost proportionately from both intracellular fluid and extracellular fluids.

15. B: When in use to deliver medications, the piggyback set should be positioned above the primary set. The secondary set is connected to the primary through the upper Y or piggyback port. The primary venous line maintains venous access when the secondary set is not in use. An extension hook is used to lower the primary set. In some cases, the secondary set may be used continuously to provide medications while the primary set maintains rate of infusion. With continuous administration, the secondary set is connected to the lower Y port.

16. A: A 1:10 dilution should be prepared to facilitate accurate dosing for doses less than 0.1 mL while a 1:100 dilution is used for doses less than 0.01 mL. Some medications are only manufactured in adult doses but are used for pediatric patients although children under 2 years should only receive medications specifically approved for children. The two-syringe technique should be used when diluting a drug. Dosages for infants and children are usually calculated according to body weight and body surface area.

17. D: The supine position leaves the toddler open and exposed and is the most likely position to frighten the child. Small children tend to curl up into a fetal position or turn away in a side-lying or prone position when they are stressed are avoiding someone, so toddlers should be placed in other positions than supine whenever possible. Lack of mobility, as with restraints, is especially stressing to a toddler who usually also has stranger anxiety and is fearful of medical staff. The preferred position is usually sitting. Toddlers are normally resistive, so whenever possible, the parent should be with the child to reduce separation anxiety.

18. D: Patients who receive multiple transfusions with citrated blood products must be carefully monitored for hypocalcemia. Calcium is important for transmitting nerve impulses and regulating muscle contraction and relaxation, including the myocardium. Calcium activates enzymes that stimulate chemical reactions and has a role in coagulation of blood. Values include:

- Normal values: 8.2 to 10.2 mg/dL.
- Hypocalcemia: <8.2 mg/dL. Critical value: <7 mg/dL.
- Hypercalcemia: >10.2 mg/dL. Critical value: >12 mg/dL.

Symptoms include tetany, tingling, seizures, altered mental status, and ventricular tachycardia. Treatment is calcium replacement and vitamin D.

19. C: Hemolytic anemia, thrombocytopenia and liver dysfunction are indications of essential fatty acid deficiency. Other indications may include dermatitis and slowed healing. Patients should

128

receive a minimum fatty acid intake of 2 to 4% of daily calories, but most patients receive 10 to 40%. Fatty acids should not exceed 60% of daily calories. Increased fatty acids (9 kcal/g) allow a decrease in glucose (3.4 kcal/g) and decrease incidence of hyperglycemia.

20. B: The dressings must be changed every 48 hours. Although transparent dressings can be left in place for 7 days, gauze dressings must be changed every 48 hours, so the schedule must correspond to the shorter time period. If Biopatch is used about an exit site, it may be left in place for 7 days, as it is antimicrobial. Dressings should be changed as needed if they loosen or become soiled to prevent skin irritation and/or infection.

21. C: The patient should be placed in Trendelenburg position (head below heart and knees flexed) to increase venous pressure and distend the subclavian vein. The neck should be hyperextended and clavicle elevated by placing a rolled towel or bolster under the back between the shoulder blades. If a jugular approach is indicated, then the patient's head should be turned in the opposite direction of the insertion point and neck extended to stabilize the vein and define the musculature.

22. B: While cultures should be done of the parenteral fluid as well as the administration set and fluid container, the method to determine if the infection is catheter-related is to culture both peripheral blood and blood drawn per the catheter to determine if the concentration of organisms is higher from blood drawn from the catheter. If catheter-related, concentration of organisms is usually five to ten times higher from the catheter-related sample than the peripheral sample.

23. A: Mitomycin, dactinomycin, and vinblastine are vesicants, which can result in severe tissue damage with blistering and ulceration of tissue. Other vesicants include idarubicin, daunorubicin, doxorubicin, mechlorethamine, mitoxantrone, vincristine, and vinorelbine. Care must be taken to avoid infiltration by use of a low-pressure infusion pump and CVC. Infusions should be started with NS. Bleomycin, carboplatin, fluorouracil, cyclophosphamide, cytarabine, and asparaginase are all non-vesicants and do not cause tissue damage. Some drugs, such as dacarbazine and streptozocin are classified as irritants, which may result in local tissue irritation.

24. D: Extravasations of plant alkaloids, such as vinblastine, are treated with recombinant hyaluronidase (such as Hylenex®). The antidote is injected in 5 small doses (0.2 mL each) about the site of extravasation. Using separate needles for each injection to avoid further irritation of the tissue. Sodium thiosulfate is used as an antidote for mechlorethamine. Totect® (dexrazoxane) is an antidote for anthracyclines, such as daunorubicin, and idarubicin. DMS0 50% solution may be used topically as an antidote to daunorubicin and doxorubicin.

25. B: The tubing is occluded by pinching above the injection port so that the nurse can aspirate for blood to ensure that the line is in place to prevent extravasation. Steps include checking to make sure the medication is compatible with the IV solution, using the port closest to the patient, cleaning the injection port, aspirating for blood, injecting the medication with the tubing clamped (timing rate of injection), and then releasing the IV tubing and checking the infusion rate.

26. B: Packed red blood cells can be refrigerated for up to 42 days or frozen for 10 years. **Platelets** can be stored up to 5 days at room temperature. **Plasma** can be frozen for one year but must be used within 24 hours after thawing. **Cryoprecipitate** can also be frozen for one year. **Granulocytes** (neutrophils) should be used as soon as possible but may be stored up to 24 hours (20-24°C) without agitation. **Lymphocytes** should be used immediately if fresh or may be frozen.

27. A: If a patient has excess hair, it should be removed by cutting with scissors or shaving with surgical clippers with disposable heads. Shaving with a razor may cause microabrasions and increase the risk of infection. Depilatory agents may be irritating to the tissue, disrupting the skin barrier. Washing the area with soap and water prior to cleansing with an antiseptic agent is indicated if the patient is excessively dirty but is not indicated simply because a patient has excess hair.

28. C: Normovolemic hemodilution involves withdrawing blood prior to surgery, replacing it with intravenous fluid to dilute the blood, and then reinfusing the blood after surgery. Usually one to two units of blood are withdrawn and simultaneously replaced with colloid or crystalloid solution. Hypervolemic hemodilution involves administering extra intravenous fluid to dilute the blood to decrease loss of blood cells with bleeding. In both cases, the purpose of diluting the blood is so that during inevitable bleeding, fewer red blood cells are lost.

29. A: Patients at risk for neutropenia should avoid fresh fruits as they may harbor organisms. Patients should also avoid fresh flowers and plants as well as people with respiratory infections or other contagious conditions and should avoid crowds. Patients must be advised to follow good hygiene and should be aware of signs of infection and the importance of checking temperature regularly. Patients are especially at risk one to two weeks after treatment when the blood count is often at its lowest point.

30. D: These symptoms are consistent with febrile nonhemolytic reaction (NHR), which occurs in about 20% of those receiving platelets. NHR is responsible for about 90% of transfusion reactions and occurs in about 10% of those who receive repeated transfusions for chronic illness. NHR occurs because some white blood cells may remain, causing the patient's antibodies to react. While patients must be carefully monitored to ensure they do not have a bacterial infection or hemolytic reaction, treatment usually involves non-aspirin antipyretics, such as acetaminophen or ibuprofen, and the transfusion resumed.

31. A: Gas bubbles present in PRBCs can indicate that bacterial infection is present. Abnormal color or cloudy appearance may indicate hemolysis is occurring. If any abnormality is noted, the blood should be returned to the laboratory and not administered. PRBCs should be initiated within 30 minutes of removal from refrigeration to prevent infection and duration of administration should not exceed 4 hours. Washed RBCs must be used within 24 hours from the beginning of the washing procedure.

32. C: If resistance is met while inserting a midline catheter in the arm, the nurse should immediately stop advancing the catheter and then change the angle of the arm or wrist and/or ask the patient to make and release a fist as this may reduce resistance. The nurse may also pull the catheter back slightly until blood returns and then slowly reinsert while flushing with NS. If these steps do not resolve the resistance, then the catheter should be removed and another site used.

33. A: Grade 1: Skin is blanched, cool with edema <1 inch from the insertion point. Pain may be present.

Grade 2: Skin is blanched, cool, with edema 1 to 6 inches from the insertion point. Pain may be present.

Grade 3: Skin is blanched, appearing almost translucent, and cool with marked edema > 6 inches from insertion point. Pain is mild to moderate.

Grade 4: Similar to grade 3 except that skin may begin to leak or become discolored and ecchymotic. Edema is deep and pitting and circulation may be impaired. Pain is moderate to severe.

34. D: In order to increase plasma volume by 1 L, 0.5 L of 25% colloid is required while 0.9% NS requires 5 to 6 liters, 3% NS requires 1.5 to 2 L, and 5% colloid requires 1 L. Colloids are protein-based and increase colloid osmotic pressure, and pull interstitial fluid into the vascular system. Crystalloids, which provide water and sodium, include NS, hypertonic saline, lactated Ringer's, D5W, and Plasma-Lyte. The volume expanding capacity correlates with sodium concentration.

35. C: These symptoms are consistent with hypokalemia, which can be caused by loop and thiazide diuretics as well as excess laxative use, vomiting, and diarrhea. Hypokalemia may also result from crash dieting, corticosteroid use, intake of large amounts of licorice as well as conditions such as hyperaldosteronism and ketoacidosis. Potassium supplements should be provided with loop and thiazide diuretics in order to maintain a normal level (3.5 to 5 mEq/L). Hyperkalemia is a level exceeding 5.5 mEq/L and hypokalemia, below 3.5 mEq/L.

36. A: Trousseau's sign is elicited by applying a blood pressure cuff to the upper arm and inflating it 20 mm Hg above systolic and leaving it in place for ≤5 minutes. A positive response occurs with increasing ischemia of the ulnar nerve: carpopedal spasm with the thumb adducted, the wrist and metacarpophalangeal joints flexed, and the interphalangeal joints extended with the fingers together. Chvostek's sign is also positive with tetany, elicited by tapping the muscles enervated by the facial nerves about 2 cm in front of the earlobe just inferior to the zygomatic arch. A positive response is twitching of the muscle.

37. D: Protamine sulfate, a heparin antagonist, is comprised of strongly basic proteins derived from salmon sperm and some other fish, so allergies to fish can put the patient at risk for protamine anaphylactic reaction. Symptoms include:

- Sudden onset of weakness, dizziness, confusion.
- Urticaria.
- Increased permeability of vascular system and loss of vascular tone.
- Severe hypotension leading to shock.
- Laryngospasm/bronchospasm with obstruction of airway causing dyspnea and wheezing.
- Nausea, vomiting, and diarrhea.
- Seizures, coma and death.

38. C: Flumazenil is a reversal agent for benzodiazepines, such as midazolam and diazepam. Flumazenil is usually given in a dose of 0.2 mg over 15 seconds and can be repeated every minute to a total of 1 mg and then at 30- to 60-minute intervals as the action of flumazenil is shorter than that of benzodiazepines. Therefore, patients must be monitored for at least 2 hours after administration to determine if further dosage is required. Naloxone should also be available as a reversal agent for opioids, such as fentanyl and meperidine.

39. B: The minimal urinary output for an adult patient is 30 mL/hr. although this level cannot be sustained for long periods, as a more normal output is 40-60 ml/hr. Minimal output for an infant or child is 0.5 mL/kg/hr. Output <30mL/0.5 mL may signal renal damage. Urinary output is influenced not only by renal status but also by hydration and medications. Vasoconstrictive medications may reduce urinary output. Patients may have low output after surgery and then diuresis as their systems clear of anesthetic drugs and other medications.

40. C: Lorazepam (Ativan®) may be administered an hour prior to treatment to reduce incidence of nausea and vomiting. In the case of severe anxiety, lorazepam may be administered intravenously as patients with anxiety are more likely to experience nausea and vomiting. Severe nausea and vomiting, which often occurs within 24 hours of treatment, may be treated with a variety of drugs, which include metoclopramide, prochlorperazine, ondansetron dexamethasone, and granisetron. Immediate treatment to control nausea and vomiting may help to alleviate future episodes, exacerbated by anticipatory anxiety.

41. B: These laboratory findings are consistent with deficient fluid volume. An increased WBC count indicating infection results from one or two cell types, but if all cell types show equal elevations, this results from concentration of the blood. Both hemoglobin and hematocrit increase as the blood volume decreases. An elevation of both BUN and creatinine indicates kidney disease, but elevated BUN alone may indicate dehydration. Serum sodium increases with dehydration. The most common cause of increased urine specific gravity is dehydration.

42. A: While at one time CVCs were routinely flushed with heparin, current recommendations are to flush with 10 mL 0.9% sodium chloride or 5% glucose as no advantage has been found to flushing with heparin, which poses risks. CVCs should be flushed before and after administration of medications as well as between different medications. Most medications are compatible with sodium chloride, but a few medications, such as amiodarone, must be flushed with 5% glucose. Some medications, such as some immunoglobulins, are incompatible with all flushing fluids, so flushing is avoided.

43. C: A volumetric pump is most appropriate for large-volume infusions with the rate controlled in mL per hour. Volumetric pumps are used for fluids and medicines that require a controlled rate of administration. A syringe pump is more appropriate for small volumes and is usually preferred for rates less than 5 mL per hour. Many specialized pumps, such as the APO-go pump (used for apomorphine) and multi-channel pumps (used to administer multiple agents at various rates) are available.

44. D: The care bundle to prevent infection from central lines includes 5 items: (1) hand hygiene and (2) using the maximum barrier precautions. Chlorhexidine (3) is recommended for skin antisepsis. The (4) subclavian vein is the preferred site for catheterization with non-tunneled catheters, but sites should be chosen to provide optimal outcomes. All lines (5) should be reviewed daily to determine if they are necessary and unnecessary lines discontinued.

45. B: Intrinsic contamination can occur at any step in the manufacturing or sterilization process. Most contamination of intravenous fluids is extrinsic and can include contamination occurring during admixture procedures, such as when a laminar flow hood is not used or improper equipment is utilized. Extrinsic contamination can also result from inadequate storage or refrigeration of use of improper techniques, such as failing to use aseptic technique when adding devices (such as filters or administration sets) or with accidental line separations. Damage to sterile containers can also result from improper handling.

46. C: A hypotonic solution, which is low in sodium, results in **ICFVE**, or "water intoxication" in which fluid moves from the vascular space to the cellular. ICFVE can also occur with administration of D5W because the glucose metabolizes quickly leaving behind hypotonic fluid. **ECFVD** can result from vomiting, diarrhea, gastrointestinal suction or fistula drainage, inadequate sodium intake and intestinal obstruction or perforated ulcer. **ECFV shift** may also occur with intestinal obstruction or perforated ulcer. **ECFVE** may result from renal disease or renal failure and heart failure because of fluid retention.

47. D: The flow rate in drops per minute is 50 to administer 1 liter of fluid over a 5-hour period. Steps to the calculations include:

- 1000 (mL) × 15 (drops/mL) = 15,000 total drops over 5 hrs
- 15,000 (drops) / 5 (hrs) = 3000 drops/hr
- 3000 (drops/hr) / 60 (min/hr) = 50 drops/min.

The Standard Drop Factor for macrodrip is 15, but some equipment has a drop factor of 10 or 20, so the nurse should always check the packaging information. The microdrip/pediatric drop factor is 60 drops/mL.

48. C: The flow rate of an intravenous solution administered per gravity is **directly proportional** to the height of the liquid column. The higher the container is, the faster the flow rate. Flow is also directly proportional to the diameter of the tubing with larger tubing resulting in faster flow. Flow is **inversely proportional** to the length of tubing, with longer tubing decreasing flow, and the viscosity of the IV fluid. PRBCs, for example, typically require a larger cannula than NS.

49. D: A severely burned adult patient may require nitrogen supplementation up to 2.5 g/kg per day because of extreme stress on the body. Nitrogen supplementation is calculated according to stress levels for those whose activity is limited. Those with no stress require 0.5 to 0.8 g/kg per day, mild stress 0.8 to 1.0, moderate, 1.0 to 1.5, and severe 1.5 to 2.0. Infants require 1.6 to 2.2 g/kg per day of nitrogen supplementation and children (over 1 year) 1.0 to 1.6 g.

50. D: The first steps to follow with a hypersensitivity reaction is to discontinue the infusion and provide rapid infusion of NS to dilute the chemotherapeutic agent. The patient's VS should be monitored and physician notified. Usually the first medication given is an antihistamine, which may be followed with corticosteroid and bronchodilator if breathing is impaired although the first drug is usually epinephrine in the case of anaphylaxis. The patient should be monitored continuously with VS and pulse oximetry until stable and then every quarter hour for up to 2 hours with life-support equipment available.

51. C: Power injectable catheters are specifically designed to accommodate contrast medium for CT. Contrast medium requires a catheter that can withstand high pressure because a standard catheter may rupture. Documentation should indicate whether catheters and ports are power injectable; and, if this cannot be verified, then a power injectable catheter should be inserted for the CT. Power injectable catheters can also tolerate higher flow rates of infusates than standard catheters.

52. B: A midline catheter can stay in place for 2-4 weeks. Catheters range in length from 7.5-20 cm and are inserted into the basilic, brachial, or cephalic veins. Areas of flexion are avoided, so the catheter can be inserted 3-5 cm above the antecubital fossa or 1-2 cm below, ensuring that the tip of the catheter is located below the axilla. Infused drugs and fluids should be in the pH range of 5-9.

53. C: Five percent dextrose in water (D5W) can safely be administered through a short peripheral catheter. Vesicants, such as vinblastine and doxorubicin, are too irritating. Isotonic fluids (D5W, NS, lactated Ringer, and Ringer's solution) can be administered but IV fluids with glucose greater than 10% (such as D20W) must be avoided. The pH of fluids should range from 5-9. Short peripheral catheters are usually inserted into the hand, wrist, or forearm.

54. B: Under the CDC's standard precautions, hand hygiene must be carried out before and after every patient contact, including touching patient, performing tasks, touching patient's immediate environment, and contact with bodily fluid. If the hands are soiled, they must be washed with soap and water instead of using alcohol-based hand cleaner. Other standard precautions include utilizing cough hygiene, and using PPE if there is possible exposure to infectious material, such as blood or other body fluids.

55. A: Chemotherapy scheduled for greater than 3 months is an indication for a CVAD. Other indications include the need for continuous infusions for a prolonged period of time (such as for parenteral nutrition), clinical instability, the need for multiple different types of infusions, the need for hemodynamic monitoring, the need for long-term intermittent therapy, and failure of peripheral venous access.

56. D: If a patient has small veins and the CRNI is unable to access a peripheral vein in the hand or forearm, the best solution is to use ultrasound to assist in accessing the vein. Feet and areas of flexion should be avoided. The ultrasound transducer can be placed transversely to the vein (vein appears as a circle) or longitudinally to the vein (vein appears as parallel lines showing upper and lower walls).

57. C: If using ultrasound guidance to locate a vein for cannulation, the CRNI can differentiate an artery from a vein because the vein compresses and the artery does not because the vein is low pressure with high volume and the artery is high pressure with low volume. Additionally, the artery pulsates, and this is evident on the ultrasound image. Arteries and veins often lie in close proximity although the artery is often deeper in the tissue.

58. A: If a patient is hypovolemic and anticipated IV replacement fluid volume is 2 to 3 L, the IV fluid that is usually the first choice is NS. However, if the patient requires large volumes of resuscitation fluids, then after the first 2 to 3 L, a switch is usually made to Lactated Ringers or Plasmalyte to avoid the patient becoming acidotic because the pH of NS is lower than that of normal blood.

59. B: D5 ½ NS is usually used for a patient that in NPO and receiving maintenance fluids preprocedure. This IV fluid provides glucose for energy as well as sodium and chloride to help to maintain electrolyte balance. D5 ½ NS contains 77 mEq/L of Na and 77 mEq/L of chloride as well as 50 mg/dL of glucose with a pH of 4.4 and 406 mOsm/L.

60. B: The *soft limit* on a smart pump refers to an alert that the CRNI can override. A *hard limit* refers to an alert that the CRNI cannot override. Smart pumps, a form of EID, contain computers and software that can be programmed to meet the individual needs of the patient; however, if information regarding dose and volume are entered manually rather than using preset parameters, the computer software will not recognize errors.

61. D: The IV fluid that is most appropriate for fluid replacement in a patient with extensive 2nd and 3rd degree burns is lactated Ringers because it most closely approximates normal blood because it contains electrolytes (Na, K, Ca, Cl, HCO₃) in a similar concentration as normal blood. With burns, extensive electrolyte loss occurs. However, lactated Ringers does not contain glucose. Plasmalyte is similar in composition.

62. B: When selecting a catheter for a PICC lime, the most appropriate catheter-to-vein ratio is equal to or less than 45%. This allows blood flow about the catheter and reduces risk of obstruction and thrombus formation. The ratio can be assessed by ultrasound prior to insertion of the catheter. Incidence of catheter-related thrombosis occurs more frequently than infections and increases risk of pulmonary embolism.

63. A: The three factors in Virchow's triad that related to catheter-associated thrombus formation are:

- Vascular injury: Injury to the vessel wall or endothelium, such as through contact with a catheter or perforation.
- Altered blood flow: Stasis, such as from inserting a catheter with a vein-to-catheter ratio greater than 45%.
- Hypercoagulability: Chemical changes in the blood that may result from medications, disease (IBD, autoimmune disorders, inherited thrombophilia), dehydration, major trauma, malignancy, infection, and surgery.

The presence of Virchow's triad increases the risk that a clot may travel to the lungs, heart, or rain, resulting in severe compromise to the patient.

64. C: If a patient with pancreatic cancer will require long-term intermittent antineoplastic chemotherapy, the recommended device is the implanted vascular access port. This is usually placed in the upper chest although a port can also be placed in the arm. When utilized for intermittent therapy, the risk of infection is lower than with other CVADs but is about the same for continuous therapy. The implanted port is easier for the patient to manage than external devices.

65. D: Chronic kidney disease is a contraindication for a PICC line because these patients are at risk for occlusion of the vessel and central vein stenosis. Additionally, the veins should be preserved as much as possible for creation of fistulas for dialysis. Other contraindications for PICC lines include burns, skin infections, or history of radiation in the insertion site, bacteremia, very small veins (<4 mm). History of major surgery distal to the insertion site (such as of the shoulder).

66. C: If taking a blood sample from a PICC line after flushing, 5 mL of blood should be withdrawn and discarded before taking the sample. Procedures may vary somewhat depending on the manufacturer's directions, but usually the PICC line is flushed with at least 10 mL NS before and after a blood draw. A heparin flush may also be required in some cases. If blood residue remains in the injection cap, the injection cap should be changed.

67. D: When therapeutic phlebotomy is utilized to treat conditions such as polycythemia vera, hemochromatosis, or porphyria, usually about 450 mL of blood is withdrawn with each treatment. This volume does not generally require replacement IV fluids, but patients should be encouraged to drink ample fluids after treatment. The frequency of therapeutic phlebotomy varies according to the severity of disease but is usually more frequent initially and decreases in frequency when the patient stabilizes.

68. C: In the chain/cycle of infection, the portal of entry link may be broken by use of face mask and gloves. The cycle/chain of infection includes the pathogen (usually bacteria or virus), reservoir (animal, human, environment), portal of exit (body fluids, wounds, respiratory system, GI system, urogenital system), mode of transmission (direct/indirect contact; contaminated food, water, or dust particles; insect bites), portal of entry (respiratory/urogenital/GI tracts and wounds), and susceptible host (human or animal).

69. D: The middle layer of the vein wall is poorly developed and has less muscle and less elastic tissue, but the lumen has a greater diameter. This allows the veins to serve as a reservoir for blood, and this is important if blood loss occurs. With blood loss, the sympathetic nervous system triggers vasoconstriction of the walls of veins, speeding the return flow of blood to the heart so that blood flow stays almost within normal parameters until about 25% of blood volume is lost.

Copyright © Mometrix Media. You have been licensed one copy of this document for personal use only. Any other reproduction or redistribution is strictly prohibited. All rights reserved.

70. A: A patient suffering from oxygen deprivation develops cyanosis because of high concentration of deoxyhemoglobin in the blood. Red cells are comprised of about 33% hemoglobin. When the hemoglobin is oxygenated, bright red oxyhemoglobin forms, but when the hemoglobin releases oxygen and is unable to become reoxygenated, the increased level of deoxyhemoglobin causes the blood to appear darker. Through the skin, blood with high levels of deoxyhemoglobin appears blue, resulting in cyanosis.

71. C: The normal pH of the blood (and the internal environment of the body) ranges from 7.35 to 7.45, making the blood slightly alkaline. A pH <7 is acidic and >7 is alkaline (basic). The pH is maintained in balance by actions of the lungs and kidneys. If a disorder in the respiratory system occurs, this can lead to respiratory acidosis or alkalosis. If a metabolic disorder occurs, this can lead to metabolic acidosis or alkalosis.

72. B: Extracellular fluids (those fluids located outside of cells) include interstitial fluids, plasma in blood vessels, and lymph in the lymphatic vessels. Extracellular fluids constitute about 37% of the volume of total body water. Intracellular fluids constitute about 63%. Blood plasma contains more protein than the other components of extracellular fluid. Extracellular fluids contain high levels of sodium, chloride, calcium, and bicarbonate ions and lower levels of other electrolytes, such as potassium, magnesium, sulfate, and phosphate.

73. D: The thirst center that regulates the sensation of thirst to maintain water balance in the body is located in the hypothalamus. As the water volume of the body decreases, the osmotic pressure of extracellular fluid increases, stimulating receptors in the hypothalamus, which responds by triggering a feeling a thirst so that the person can increase the intake of fluids. Thirst is usually triggered when the water volume decreases by about 1%. Receptors in the stomach send messages to the hypothalamus that fluid intake has occurred, and the hypothalamus, in turn, inhibits the sensation of thirst.

74. D: After a patient receives a hazardous drug, such as an antineoplastic agent, the CRNI should use extra precautions when handling or exposed to the patient's bodily fluids for 48 hours. Extra precautions include wearing double chemotherapy gloves (which are thicker than ordinary treatment gloves) and a disposable gown. If possible, disposable linens should be used and placed in a leakproof bag for contaminants for disposal.

75. B: If a patient has a large wound infected with MRSA, contact precautions are indicated. Standard precautions are indicated for all patients and are included in contact precautions. Other conditions for which contact precautions are indicated include enteric pathogens, _Clostridium difficile_, bronchiolitis, croup, and other resistant organisms. Varicella requires both contact and airborne precautions.

76. A: The preferred vein for venipuncture to obtain a blood sample with the H-shaped vein distribution pattern is generally the median cubital vein. The three veins that are evident in about 70% of people form an H-shape and include the median cubital vein, the cephalic vein (the second choice), and the basilic vein. In the M-shaped pattern, the three veins include the intermediate antebrachial vein, the intermediate cephalic vein, and the intermediate basilic vein.

77. B: While the basilic vein is usually easy to palpate because it is large, it tends to roll easily and this can result in accidental puncture of the medial cutaneous nerve or the brachial artery because they lie in close proximity to the vein. Whether the vein distribution pattern is H-shaped or M-shaped, the basilic vein is the last choice for venipuncture. Additionally, venipuncture of this vein is more painful that of the other veins.

78. C: According to the order of the draw established by the CLSI, the blood sample that would be obtained first is the sterile tube (blood culture). This is followed in order by the blue-top coagulation tube, the serum tube, the heparin tube with/without gel plasma separator, the EDTA tube, and the glycolytic tube. The tubes according to color begin with yellow, then light blue, then red, green lavender, pink pearl top, and gray.

79. A: If preparing an IV infusion of a chemotherapeutic agent that has splash potential, the PPE that is required includes double gloves, gown, and eye protection. Respiratory protection is only indicated if the drug also has the potential for inhalation. When opening an ampule, double gloves, gown, and eye and respiratory protection must be utilized. NIOSH classifies chemotherapeutic agents as hazardous drugs because of their carcinogenicity, teratogenicity, reproductive toxicity, organ toxicity and genotoxicity.

80. A: If, when preparing a chemotherapeutic agent for IV infusion, the CRNI accidentally spills approximately 10 mL of the drug in the safety cabinet, the first step is to utilize the spill kit to contain the drug. A spill kit should always be readily available. Because the spill exceeds 5 mL, an accident report must be filed and the safety director notified. If the spill had occurred outside of the safety cabinet, then all people must be cleared from the area and absorbent pads placed over the spill. The pads are then placed in a hazardous waste container and the area cleansed with soap and water.

81. B: One mL of blood is usually needed for ABB analysis. If ABG analysis must be repeated frequently, then sites should be alternated to reduce incidence of complications, such as hematoma and scarring of the artery. An arterial line may be used to obtain samples as well. An ABG should not be obtained from an artery if there is infection, no palpable pulse, negative Modified Allen test, or arterial grafts.

82. D: The level of potassium increases in stored blood (especially if stored for more than 12 days), and this can result in hyperkalemia in patients following multiple blood transfusions. Additionally, as red blood cells break down, this releases potassium. Patients who are hypovolemic before receiving transfusions are at increased risk of developing hyperkalemia. Absorption filters may be utilized when administering PRBCs to decrease potassium in the transfusion.

83. B: Type II hypersensitivity reaction is associated with blood transfusion incompatibility reactions. Cytotoxic response occurs when the body produces antibodies to body constituents, such as the surface of red blood cells. The response is mediated by IgM and IgG. The complement cascade is implemented and produces biochemicals that destroy the antigen-bearing cells. This type of hypersensitivity reaction occurs within minutes or hours. Patients may experience hemolytic anemia, pulmonary failure, and/or renal failure.

84. C: The IV administration of an immediate-use compounded sterile product (CSP) must be initiated within 60 minutes. Immediate-use CSPs include medications that are required for emergent situations as well as those that remain stable for a short period of time. Immediate-use CSPs cannot contain more than three components, including the diluent. If the immediate-use CSP cannot be used within 60 minutes, then the product must be properly discarded. The label must contain patient ID, names and amounts of ingredients, name/initial of the preparer, and the exact time and date by which the immediate-use CSP must be administered.

85. D: A short 5 cm catheter length is associated with shorter catheter survival time while the longer 12 cm catheter is associated with longer catheter survival time. The diameter of the vein appears to have no effect on survival time, but depths of 1.2 cm or more shorten survival time as does insertion of catheters into deep brachial or basilic veins. Using ultrasound decreases the number of attempts needed to insert the catheter and decreases the risk of catheter failure.

86. A: Near-infrared (nIR) light devices are appropriate to aid in cannulation of superficial peripheral veins. The insertion site is illuminated by the device, which projects an image of the veins on the skin or onto a screen, making it easier to locate a suitable vein. The nIR device may also be used for radial artery cannulation in pediatric patients. The light penetrates the tissue, and the rate of absorption is different between soft tissue and blood, which causes the veins to illuminate.

87. D: The type of needle that must be used to access an implanted CVA port is the Huber needle, which is a hollow non-coring needle with a long, tapered point that can penetrate the port without causing damage or removing any silicone (which could cause obstruction) from the port. Most ports can withstand up to about 2000 punctures. Huber needles are available in various sizes (19-24) and at various lengths. The needles may be straight or have a 90-degree angle.

88. B: If using the Vein Entry Indicator Device (VEID), the device indicates penetration of a vein by beeping. The device is attached to the catheter needle insertion set and senses a change in pressure as the needle enters the vein. The beeping begins within a tenth of a second of insertion and stops when the needle is withdrawn from the vein. This device is indicated for patients with hard to locate veins.

89. A: For a CVAD with an upper body insertion site, the tip should be located near the superior cavoatrial junction, where the superior vena cava and the right atrium meet. If the tip is positioned further into the right atrium, such as near the tricuspid valve, or into the right ventricle, it can cause cardiac dysrhythmias. Some type of imaging technology should be utilized to ensure proper tip placement.

90. A: In order to utilize ECG tip confirmation for insertion of a CVAD, P waves must be present, so conditions that may affect the P wave, such as severe tachycardia, AF, and AFL, require other methods to ensure proper tip placement, such as post-procedure chest x-ray or insertion of the CVAD under fluoroscopy. With ECG placement, the P wave elevates as the tip reaches the superior vena cava and moves toward the right atrium.

91. B: If vesicant (anthracycline) extravasation occurs, the CRNI should immediately stop the infusion and aspirate any residual vesicant from the needle or catheter. Vesicants, such as anthracyclines, are especially toxic to the tissues and may cause blistering and ulceration. Cold compresses may be applied to relieve discomfort and swelling, and antidotes, such as hyaluronidase, may be injected subcutaneously into the tissue to reduce reaction. If hyaluronidase is used, then warm compresses should be applied to increase circulation.

92. D: A blood warmer can be used with red blood cells. However, platelets, granulocytes, and cryoprecipitate should not be warmed as this may make them less effective. Only FDA approved blood warmers should be utilized and testing should include ensuring temperature and temperature alarms are functioning properly. Generally, blood warmers only raise the temperature of the blood to 33-36 °C when delivered at a rapid flow rate.

93. C: While all of these may be of some concern, the nurse should be especially on alert for hypovolemia in a patient undergoing plasmapheresis/therapeutic plasma exchange because about 15% of the patient's blood volume is out of the body and being processed during the procedure. Plasmapheresis/therapeutic plasma exchange removes some components of the plasma and then reinfuses the remaining plasma and additional fluid (such as albumin) into the patient. The patient must be carefully monitored for hypotension and any indication of reaction, such as fever, headache, and chills.

94. A: When administering platelets to a patient, the infusion should be done as fast as the patient can tolerate because platelets tend to clump together if the transfusion takes too long. Platelet concentrate is usually about 50 mL. Platelet transfusions may be given for leukemia, other malignancies, and severe thrombocytopenia. While ABO/Rh compatibility is desired, the number of red blood cells that remain is usually too low to cause a reaction although Rh antibodies may form if the patient is Rh-.

95. C: The basic maintenance fluid requirement for parenteral formulations for the first 20 kg of weight for adults is 30 to 35 mL/kg/d. Above 20 kg, 20 mL is added for each kilogram. This basic maintenance fluid requirement may need to be adjusted upward if the patient is losing significant fluids, such as through diarrhea or other fluid loss, or adjusted downward if the patient is retaining fluids.

96. D: When using a primary infusion set with a secondary (piggyback) set, the purpose of the check valve is to prevent retrograde flow of the solution. The check valve is a Y connector that joins the primary infusion tubing with the piggyback tubing. The check valve allows fluids in the piggyback tubing to flow in only one direction.

97. C: A secondary (piggyback) administration set can deliver up to 500 mL. The secondary administration set attaches to the primary administration in order to administer a limited amount of fluid and medication. The drop factor ranges from 10 to 20 drops per mL. When administering fluid/medications from the piggyback container, the primary infusion container is positioned lower than the piggyback container.

98. B: A risk especially associated with the use of a primary Y administration set is air embolism. A primary Y infusion set joins two primary infusion sets, each with a separate drip chamber and clamp, and allows for the fluids to intermix and large volumes of liquids to be administered rapidly; however, air can be drawn into an administration set if a container should empty completely.

99. A: If a patient with hyperemesis gravidarum has an order for IV dextrose solution because of hypoglycemia and dehydration, the CRNI should verify that the patient has received thiamine before the IV. HG is usually treated with NS because dextrose solutions may trigger Wernicke's encephalopathy, but thiamine may prevent this disorder.

100. C: With a needleless connector with positive fluid displacement, it is important to clamp the catheter after disconnection. Needless connectors may be simple or complex, and some may have negative fluid displacement (which requires that pressure be continued with the syringe used to flush while clamping the catheter). A needleless connector with neutral displacement allows the catheter to be clamped either before or after disconnection.

101. B: The type of filter would be appropriate for reinfusion of autologous blood retrieved during surgery involving extensive blood loss is the microaggregate filter. Microaggregates are small particles (platelets, nonviable leukocytes, and strands of fibrin). Standard clot filters allow microaggregates to pass through. Leukocyte reduction filters are used to remove leukocytes from RBCs and platelets.

102. D: The most common type of CVAD is the PICC. The PICC insertion site is usually placed distal to the antecubital fossa and may be single lumen or multiple lumen. PICC lines are typically 50 to 60 cm long and available in various gauges. PICC lines may be used for short term therapy or long-term therapy up to 12 months.

103. A: When receiving IV fluids, older adults are most at risk for hypervolemic hyponatremia. As a result of aging, older adults are less able to excrete water and dilute urine because they have fewer effective nephrons and decreased renal blood flow. Thus, older adults tend to retain fluid when receiving intravenous fluids, especially if they receive excessive fluids for their needs.

104. B: Femoral catheters for vascular access for hemodialysis should be left in place for no longer than 5 days. Femoral catheters are generally contraindicated because of the increased potential for complications and infections and should only be utilized for short periods for patients who are bedbound. While puncture of the femoral artery usually only results in a hematoma, with femoral access, dialysis should be heparin-free for at least the first 24 hours. Femoral access increases risk of vein thrombosis.

105. D: In order to reduce the risk of CLABSI from non-tunneled CVADs in adults, the preferred vein is the subclavian although this may pose increased risk of stenosis and occlusion in patients with chronic kidney disease. Non-tunneled CVADs are used primarily for short term CVA in acute care patients. Catheters may be single to quadruple lumen. Risks include air embolism, infection, and pneumothorax.

106. A: If using a use-activated container to administer an IV drug, it is essential that the CRNI ensure complete rupture of the reservoir. The use-activated container has two compartments: One compartment contains a solution (such as D5W or NS) and the other compartment contains a medication and diluent. Pressure must be applied to the container to rupture the diaphragm separating the components, allowing them to mix for administration.

107. C: The *occlusion alarm* on the EID indicates the fluid is not flowing either from the container to the pump or from the pump to the patient. The *air-in-line alarm* detects air somewhere in the tubing. The *infusion complete alarm* sounds when the container is nearing empty to avoid a dry container. The *low battery alarm* indicates a need to replace batteries or connect to a power source. The *nonfunctional alarm* indicates that the pump is not working correctly, and the patient must be disconnected from the EID.

108. B: When preparing a patient for insertion of a tunneled catheter into the internal jugular vein, the patient should be placed in 10-15° Trendelenburg. This Trendelenburg position allows the internal jugular vein to distend, making it easier to see, and reduced the risk of air embolism. A child's head should be turned to the opposite side, but an adult's head may be maintained in neutral position.

109. D: If a patient is receiving total parenteral nutrition (TPN), fat emulsions should generally not provide more than 30% of total energy requirement and not exceed a maximum dose of 2.5 g/kg/d. A total nutrient admixture that contains fat emulsion, dextrose, and amino acids is widely used although fat emulsion may be administered separately. Commercially-prepared TPN solutions contain dextrose and protein (amino acids), but electrolytes, vitamins, and trace elements are individualized.

110. A: Trace mineral deficiencies associated with TPN include:

- *Zinc*: Dermatitis, hair loss, anorexia, immunocompromise, stomatitis, glossitis, depressed healing.
- *Chromium*: Hyperlipidemia, glucose intolerance, neuropathy

- *Copper*: Peripheral numbness, weakness, ataxia, leukopenia, anemia (hypochromatic, microcytic, normocytic).
- *Manganese*: Weight loss, dermatitis.
- *Selenium*: Depigmentation, muscle soreness/myopathy, cardiomyopathy, anemia (macrocytic).

111. B: If the CRNI is unable to insert an IV to provide fluids into a child dehydrated from diarrhea, the best alternative is likely hypodermoclysis. A small gauge needle or angiocath is inserted into subcutaneous tissue of the lateral abdomen or inner or outer aspect of the thigh. The fluids absorb quickly. Administration per gravity is often preferred because the flow normally slows when the tissues are filled with fluids. Flow rate is generally 20 ml/kg over the course of an hour.

112. D: If administering infusate in a glass container, a vented administration set is required so that air can enter the container as the fluid flows out because the glass container does not collapse as do the pliable plastic containers. While the glass containers are clear and it is easy to assess the contents for clarity, the container can break easily, and coring may occur with puncture of the stopper.

113. C: With CRBSI, the source of the infection is always the catheter itself, so it is a more limited diagnosis that CLABSI, which may be associated with various intrinsic factors (such as hematologic spread from distant infection) and extrinsic factors (such as skin organisms and contaminated infusate). CRBSI is the greatest risk factor for the development of healthcare-associated infections, such as bacteremia and sepsis. Diagnosis is per blood culture and culture of the tip of the catheter.

114. D: When a child is utilizing patient-controlled analgesia (PCA), the limit (total dosage that can be delivered in a set duration of time) is usually set at 4 hours. The PCA must be reset every 4 hours to ensure that the patient's use of medication is monitored, to avoid the chance of overdose, and to respond to changes in condition and changing need for medication. The lockout interval is the time required between dosages. The PCA may deliver boluses or continuous infusion.

115. A: The primary use for peristaltic pumps is for enteral feedings. *Peristaltic pumps* act by applying intermittent pressure to the tubing, an action similar to milking the tube, which moves the fluid through the tubing. *Volumetric pumps*, on the other hand, use a reservoir and monitor the displacement of fluid during fill and empty cycles. *Syringe pumps* use a syringe as the container, usually to deliver small doses of medication.

116. B: Lipid-based solutions should be avoided with plastic administration sets that include DEHP (a plasticizer that makes the sets pliable). DEHP is found in many types of polyvinyl chloride tubing. However, DEHP is a toxin that can be leached from containers by drugs (such as some chemotherapeutic agents) and by lipid-based solutions. Lipid-solutions are typically supplied in glass containers with vented administration sets. Non-DEHP plastic containers are available as well.

117. A: The preferred vascular access device for patients with chronic kidney disease is the AV fistula followed by the AV graft and the long-term VAD. The AV fistula is the recommended access for hemodialysis because it is the longest lasting and tends to have a lower risk of blood clotting. Use of the patient's own vessels is preferred. One problem with the AV fistula is that it can take one to four months to mature, during which an alternate access is required.

118. C: If using a transillumination device, such as the Venoscope®, the first thing that the CRNI should do when a dark line appears between the arms of the device is to apply pressure to both arms of the device and observe the dark line. The pressure should cause the line to disappear and releasing the pressure should cause it to reappear, indicating that it is a vein. Then, the outline of the vein can be traced with a surgical marking pen or the device secured with Velcro bands and then the needle inserted.

119. A: Overfeeding (excessive caloric intake) is associated with increased risk of infection with total parenteral nutrition (TPN). One of the most frequent serious complication of TPN is sepsis, so patients must be monitored very carefully. Overfeeding may exacerbate hyperglycemia, and high levels of blood glucose (≥165) are also associated with increased risk of infection. Older adults, and patients that are very small or very large have increased risk of overfeeding. Excessive caloric intake may result in hyperglycemia, fatty liver, and hypertriglyceridemia.

120. D: An EID is unable to detect infiltration, so the infusion site should be checked frequently and the patient advised to notify a nurse if signs or symptoms of infiltration occur, such as edema about insertion site, pain, and sensation of cold where the infusate leaks into the tissues. For infiltration, the infusion must be stopped immediately and the needle or catheter removed.

How to Overcome Test Anxiety

Just the thought of taking a test is enough to make most people a little nervous. A test is an important event that can have a long-term impact on your future, so it's important to take it seriously and it's natural to feel anxious about performing well. But just because anxiety is normal, that doesn't mean that it's helpful in test taking, or that you should simply accept it as part of your life. Anxiety can have a variety of effects. These effects can be mild, like making you feel slightly nervous, or severe, like blocking your ability to focus or remember even a simple detail.

If you experience test anxiety—whether severe or mild—it's important to know how to beat it. To discover this, first you need to understand what causes test anxiety.

Causes of Test Anxiety

While we often think of anxiety as an uncontrollable emotional state, it can actually be caused by simple, practical things. One of the most common causes of test anxiety is that a person does not feel adequately prepared for their test. This feeling can be the result of many different issues such as poor study habits or lack of organization, but the most common culprit is time management. Starting to study too late, failing to organize your study time to cover all of the material, or being distracted while you study will mean that you're not well prepared for the test. This may lead to cramming the night before, which will cause you to be physically and mentally exhausted for the test. Poor time management also contributes to feelings of stress, fear, and hopelessness as you realize you are not well prepared but don't know what to do about it.

Other times, test anxiety is not related to your preparation for the test but comes from unresolved fear. This may be a past failure on a test, or poor performance on tests in general. It may come from comparing yourself to others who seem to be performing better or from the stress of living up to expectations. Anxiety may be driven by fears of the future—how failure on this test would affect your educational and career goals. These fears are often completely irrational, but they can still negatively impact your test performance.

> **Review Video: 3 Reasons You Have Test Anxiety**
> Visit mometrix.com/academy and enter code: 428468

Elements of Test Anxiety

As mentioned earlier, test anxiety is considered to be an emotional state, but it has physical and mental components as well. Sometimes you may not even realize that you are suffering from test anxiety until you notice the physical symptoms. These can include trembling hands, rapid heartbeat, sweating, nausea, and tense muscles. Extreme anxiety may lead to fainting or vomiting. Obviously, any of these symptoms can have a negative impact on testing. It is important to recognize them as soon as they begin to occur so that you can address the problem before it damages your performance.

> **Review Video: 3 Ways to Tell You Have Test Anxiety**
> Visit mometrix.com/academy and enter code: 927847

The mental components of test anxiety include trouble focusing and inability to remember learned information. During a test, your mind is on high alert, which can help you recall information and stay focused for an extended period of time. However, anxiety interferes with your mind's natural processes, causing you to blank out, even on the questions you know well. The strain of testing during anxiety makes it difficult to stay focused, especially on a test that may take several hours. Extreme anxiety can take a huge mental toll, making it difficult not only to recall test information but even to understand the test questions or pull your thoughts together.

> **Review Video: How Test Anxiety Affects Memory**
> Visit mometrix.com/academy and enter code: 609003

Effects of Test Anxiety

Test anxiety is like a disease—if left untreated, it will get progressively worse. Anxiety leads to poor performance, and this reinforces the feelings of fear and failure, which in turn lead to poor performances on subsequent tests. It can grow from a mild nervousness to a crippling condition. If allowed to progress, test anxiety can have a big impact on your schooling, and consequently on your future.

Test anxiety can spread to other parts of your life. Anxiety on tests can become anxiety in any stressful situation, and blanking on a test can turn into panicking in a job situation. But fortunately, you don't have to let anxiety rule your testing and determine your grades. There are a number of relatively simple steps you can take to move past anxiety and function normally on a test and in the rest of life.

> **Review Video: How Test Anxiety Impacts Your Grades**
> Visit mometrix.com/academy and enter code: 939819

Physical Steps for Beating Test Anxiety

While test anxiety is a serious problem, the good news is that it can be overcome. It doesn't have to control your ability to think and remember information. While it may take time, you can begin taking steps today to beat anxiety.

Just as your first hint that you may be struggling with anxiety comes from the physical symptoms, the first step to treating it is also physical. Rest is crucial for having a clear, strong mind. If you are tired, it is much easier to give in to anxiety. But if you establish good sleep habits, your body and mind will be ready to perform optimally, without the strain of exhaustion. Additionally, sleeping well helps you to retain information better, so you're more likely to recall the answers when you see the test questions.

Getting good sleep means more than going to bed on time. It's important to allow your brain time to relax. Take study breaks from time to time so it doesn't get overworked, and don't study right before bed. Take time to rest your mind before trying to rest your body, or you may find it difficult to fall asleep.

> **Review Video: The Importance of Sleep for Your Brain**
> Visit mometrix.com/academy and enter code: 319338

Along with sleep, other aspects of physical health are important in preparing for a test. Good nutrition is vital for good brain function. Sugary foods and drinks may give a burst of energy but this burst is followed by a crash, both physically and emotionally. Instead, fuel your body with protein and vitamin-rich foods.

Also, drink plenty of water. Dehydration can lead to headaches and exhaustion, especially if your brain is already under stress from the rigors of the test. Particularly if your test is a long one, drink water during the breaks. And if possible, take an energy-boosting snack to eat between sections.

> **Review Video: How Diet Can Affect your Mood**
> Visit mometrix.com/academy and enter code: 624317

Along with sleep and diet, a third important part of physical health is exercise. Maintaining a steady workout schedule is helpful, but even taking 5-minute study breaks to walk can help get your blood pumping faster and clear your head. Exercise also releases endorphins, which contribute to a positive feeling and can help combat test anxiety.

When you nurture your physical health, you are also contributing to your mental health. If your body is healthy, your mind is much more likely to be healthy as well. So take time to rest, nourish your body with healthy food and water, and get moving as much as possible. Taking these physical steps will make you stronger and more able to take the mental steps necessary to overcome test anxiety.

> **Review Video: How to Stay Healthy and Prevent Test Anxiety**
> Visit mometrix.com/academy and enter code: 877894

Mental Steps for Beating Test Anxiety

Working on the mental side of test anxiety can be more challenging, but as with the physical side, there are clear steps you can take to overcome it. As mentioned earlier, test anxiety often stems from lack of preparation, so the obvious solution is to prepare for the test. Effective studying may be the most important weapon you have for beating test anxiety, but you can and should employ several other mental tools to combat fear.

First, boost your confidence by reminding yourself of past success—tests or projects that you aced. If you're putting as much effort into preparing for this test as you did for those, there's no reason you should expect to fail here. Work hard to prepare; then trust your preparation.

Second, surround yourself with encouraging people. It can be helpful to find a study group, but be sure that the people you're around will encourage a positive attitude. If you spend time with others who are anxious or cynical, this will only contribute to your own anxiety. Look for others who are motivated to study hard from a desire to succeed, not from a fear of failure.

Third, reward yourself. A test is physically and mentally tiring, even without anxiety, and it can be helpful to have something to look forward to. Plan an activity following the test, regardless of the outcome, such as going to a movie or getting ice cream.

When you are taking the test, if you find yourself beginning to feel anxious, remind yourself that you know the material. Visualize successfully completing the test. Then take a few deep, relaxing breaths and return to it. Work through the questions carefully but with confidence, knowing that you are capable of succeeding.

Developing a healthy mental approach to test taking will also aid in other areas of life. Test anxiety affects more than just the actual test—it can be damaging to your mental health and even contribute to depression. It's important to beat test anxiety before it becomes a problem for more than testing.

> **Review Video: Test Anxiety and Depression**
> Visit mometrix.com/academy and enter code: 904704

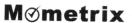

Study Strategy

Being prepared for the test is necessary to combat anxiety, but what does being prepared look like? You may study for hours on end and still not feel prepared. What you need is a strategy for test prep. The next few pages outline our recommended steps to help you plan out and conquer the challenge of preparation.

STEP 1: SCOPE OUT THE TEST

Learn everything you can about the format (multiple choice, essay, etc.) and what will be on the test. Gather any study materials, course outlines, or sample exams that may be available. Not only will this help you to prepare, but knowing what to expect can help to alleviate test anxiety.

STEP 2: MAP OUT THE MATERIAL

Look through the textbook or study guide and make note of how many chapters or sections it has. Then divide these over the time you have. For example, if a book has 15 chapters and you have five days to study, you need to cover three chapters each day. Even better, if you have the time, leave an extra day at the end for overall review after you have gone through the material in depth.

If time is limited, you may need to prioritize the material. Look through it and make note of which sections you think you already have a good grasp on, and which need review. While you are studying, skim quickly through the familiar sections and take more time on the challenging parts. Write out your plan so you don't get lost as you go. Having a written plan also helps you feel more in control of the study, so anxiety is less likely to arise from feeling overwhelmed at the amount to cover.

STEP 3: GATHER YOUR TOOLS

Decide what study method works best for you. Do you prefer to highlight in the book as you study and then go back over the highlighted portions? Or do you type out notes of the important information? Or is it helpful to make flashcards that you can carry with you? Assemble the pens, index cards, highlighters, post-it notes, and any other materials you may need so you won't be distracted by getting up to find things while you study.

If you're having a hard time retaining the information or organizing your notes, experiment with different methods. For example, try color-coding by subject with colored pens, highlighters, or post-it notes. If you learn better by hearing, try recording yourself reading your notes so you can listen while in the car, working out, or simply sitting at your desk. Ask a friend to quiz you from your flashcards, or try teaching someone the material to solidify it in your mind.

STEP 4: CREATE YOUR ENVIRONMENT

It's important to avoid distractions while you study. This includes both the obvious distractions like visitors and the subtle distractions like an uncomfortable chair (or a too-comfortable couch that makes you want to fall asleep). Set up the best study environment possible: good lighting and a comfortable work area. If background music helps you focus, you may want to turn it on, but otherwise keep the room quiet. If you are using a computer to take notes, be sure you don't have any other windows open, especially applications like social media, games, or anything else that could distract you. Silence your phone and turn off notifications. Be sure to keep water close by so you stay hydrated while you study (but avoid unhealthy drinks and snacks).

Also, take into account the best time of day to study. Are you freshest first thing in the morning? Try to set aside some time then to work through the material. Is your mind clearer in the afternoon or evening? Schedule your study session then. Another method is to study at the same time of day that you will take the test, so that your brain gets used to working on the material at that time and will be ready to focus at test time.

STEP 5: STUDY!

Once you have done all the study preparation, it's time to settle into the actual studying. Sit down, take a few moments to settle your mind so you can focus, and begin to follow your study plan. Don't give in to distractions or let yourself procrastinate. This is your time to prepare so you'll be ready to fearlessly approach the test. Make the most of the time and stay focused.

Of course, you don't want to burn out. If you study too long you may find that you're not retaining the information very well. Take regular study breaks. For example, taking five minutes out of every hour to walk briskly, breathing deeply and swinging your arms, can help your mind stay fresh.

As you get to the end of each chapter or section, it's a good idea to do a quick review. Remind yourself of what you learned and work on any difficult parts. When you feel that you've mastered the material, move on to the next part. At the end of your study session, briefly skim through your notes again.

But while review is helpful, cramming last minute is NOT. If at all possible, work ahead so that you won't need to fit all your study into the last day. Cramming overloads your brain with more information than it can process and retain, and your tired mind may struggle to recall even previously learned information when it is overwhelmed with last-minute study. Also, the urgent nature of cramming and the stress placed on your brain contribute to anxiety. You'll be more likely to go to the test feeling unprepared and having trouble thinking clearly.

So don't cram, and don't stay up late before the test, even just to review your notes at a leisurely pace. Your brain needs rest more than it needs to go over the information again. In fact, plan to finish your studies by noon or early afternoon the day before the test. Give your brain the rest of the day to relax or focus on other things, and get a good night's sleep. Then you will be fresh for the test and better able to recall what you've studied.

STEP 6: TAKE A PRACTICE TEST

Many courses offer sample tests, either online or in the study materials. This is an excellent resource to check whether you have mastered the material, as well as to prepare for the test format and environment.

Check the test format ahead of time: the number of questions, the type (multiple choice, free response, etc.), and the time limit. Then create a plan for working through them. For example, if you have 30 minutes to take a 60-question test, your limit is 30 seconds per question. Spend less time on the questions you know well so that you can take more time on the difficult ones.

If you have time to take several practice tests, take the first one open book, with no time limit. Work through the questions at your own pace and make sure you fully understand them. Gradually work up to taking a test under test conditions: sit at a desk with all study materials put away and set a timer. Pace yourself to make sure you finish the test with time to spare and go back to check your answers if you have time.

After each test, check your answers. On the questions you missed, be sure you understand why you missed them. Did you misread the question (tests can use tricky wording)? Did you forget the information? Or was it something you hadn't learned? Go back and study any shaky areas that the practice tests reveal.

Taking these tests not only helps with your grade, but also aids in combating test anxiety. If you're already used to the test conditions, you're less likely to worry about it, and working through tests until you're scoring well gives you a confidence boost. Go through the practice tests until you feel comfortable, and then you can go into the test knowing that you're ready for it.

Test Tips

On test day, you should be confident, knowing that you've prepared well and are ready to answer the questions. But aside from preparation, there are several test day strategies you can employ to maximize your performance.

First, as stated before, get a good night's sleep the night before the test (and for several nights before that, if possible). Go into the test with a fresh, alert mind rather than staying up late to study.

Try not to change too much about your normal routine on the day of the test. It's important to eat a nutritious breakfast, but if you normally don't eat breakfast at all, consider eating just a protein bar. If you're a coffee drinker, go ahead and have your normal coffee. Just make sure you time it so that the caffeine doesn't wear off right in the middle of your test. Avoid sugary beverages, and drink enough water to stay hydrated but not so much that you need a restroom break 10 minutes into the test. If your test isn't first thing in the morning, consider going for a walk or doing a light workout before the test to get your blood flowing.

Allow yourself enough time to get ready, and leave for the test with plenty of time to spare so you won't have the anxiety of scrambling to arrive in time. Another reason to be early is to select a good seat. It's helpful to sit away from doors and windows, which can be distracting. Find a good seat, get out your supplies, and settle your mind before the test begins.

When the test begins, start by going over the instructions carefully, even if you already know what to expect. Make sure you avoid any careless mistakes by following the directions.

Then begin working through the questions, pacing yourself as you've practiced. If you're not sure on an answer, don't spend too much time on it, and don't let it shake your confidence. Either skip it and come back later, or eliminate as many wrong answers as possible and guess among the remaining ones. Don't dwell on these questions as you continue—put them out of your mind and focus on what lies ahead.

Be sure to read all of the answer choices, even if you're sure the first one is the right answer. Sometimes you'll find a better one if you keep reading. But don't second-guess yourself if you do immediately know the answer. Your gut instinct is usually right. Don't let test anxiety rob you of the information you know.

If you have time at the end of the test (and if the test format allows), go back and review your answers. Be cautious about changing any, since your first instinct tends to be correct, but make sure you didn't misread any of the questions or accidentally mark the wrong answer choice. Look over any you skipped and make an educated guess.

At the end, leave the test feeling confident. You've done your best, so don't waste time worrying about your performance or wishing you could change anything. Instead, celebrate the successful

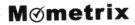

completion of this test. And finally, use this test to learn how to deal with anxiety even better next time.

> **Review Video: <u>5 Tips to Beat Test Anxiety</u>**
> Visit mometrix.com/academy and enter code: 570656

Important Qualification

Not all anxiety is created equal. If your test anxiety is causing major issues in your life beyond the classroom or testing center, or if you are experiencing troubling physical symptoms related to your anxiety, it may be a sign of a serious physiological or psychological condition. If this sounds like your situation, we strongly encourage you to seek professional help.

150

Thank You

We at Mometrix would like to extend our heartfelt thanks to you, our friend and patron, for allowing us to play a part in your journey. It is a privilege to serve people from all walks of life who are unified in their commitment to building the best future they can for themselves.

The preparation you devote to these important testing milestones may be the most valuable educational opportunity you have for making a real difference in your life. We encourage you to put your heart into it—that feeling of succeeding, overcoming, and yes, conquering will be well worth the hours you've invested.

We want to hear your story, your struggles and your successes, and if you see any opportunities for us to improve our materials so we can help others even more effectively in the future, please share that with us as well. **The team at Mometrix would be absolutely thrilled to hear from you!** So please, send us an email (support@mometrix.com) and let's stay in touch.

> **If you'd like some additional help, check out these other resources we offer for your exam:**
> **http://mometrixflashcards.com/CRNI**

Additional Bonus Material

Due to our efforts to try to keep this book to a manageable length, we've created a link that will give you access to all of your additional bonus material.

Please visit https://www.mometrix.com/bonus948/crni to access the information.